ENGINES OF EMPOWERMENT

Using
Information Technology
to Create
Healthy Communities
and Challenge
Public Policy

ENGINES OF EMPOWERMENT

Using Information Technology to Create Healthy Communities and Challenge Public Policy

NANCY MILIO

Health Administration Press
Chicago, Illinois 1996

00 99 98 97 96 5 4 3 2 1

Library of Congress Cataloging-in-Publication Data

Milio, Nancy.

Engines of empowerment : using information technology to create healthy communities and challenge public policy / Nancy Milio.
p. cm.
Includes bibliographical references and index.
ISBN 1-56793-038-7 (softbound : alk. paper)
1. Community health services. 2. Information technology. 3. Medical policy. 4. Poor—Medical care. 5. Health promotion.
I. Title.
[DNLM: 1. Community Health Services—trends—United States. 2. Information Systems. 3. Public Policy—United States. 4. Social Support. WA 546 AA1 M58e 1996]
RA425.M485 1996 362.1'2—dc20 95–43993 CIP

The paper used in this publication meets the minimum requirements of American National Standard for Information Sciences—Permanence of Paper for Printed Library Materials, ANSI Z39.48–1984. ♾ ™

Health Administration Press
A division of the Foundation of the
American College of Healthcare Executives
One North Franklin Street
Chicago, IL 60606
312/424–2800

CONTENTS

PREFACE

These engines of mischief were sentenced to die
By unanimous vote of the trade
and Ludd who can all opposition defy
Was the grand executioner made.

Let the haughty no longer the humble oppress
Then shall Ludd sheath his conquering sword,
His grievances instantly meet with redress
Then peace will be quickly restored.

Nineteenth-century Luddite song quoted in
E. P. Thompson,
The Making of the English Working Class

TEN YEARS ago, I was somewhat like the folk long ago who decried the machines of the emerging Industrial Revolution, a computer Luddite of sorts. I was concerned about the negative social consequences of the new electronic information technology, especially among less advantaged groups. I still am. However, after a decade of learning, I am more aware not only of the inexorable movement toward the electronic future, but also of the possibilities these tools have to benefit less favored groups and communities.

But possible and desired futures do not just "happen" in a world where big governments and big corporations compete and collaborate. The path to the future is being shaped by human choice. The prime mover will be the aggressive search for markets; or perhaps enlightened public policy that will give some priority to equity over market control. The priorities that will guide massive developmental resources are being set by negotiation among public policymakers and others who are at the table. The future and its social consequences are being shaped by the groups who can get to the table and make their voices heard.

This book will present and demonstrate the contexts, possibilities, perspectives, and prospects for electronic futures, giving priority to the paths that might best help lead to greater well-being, health, and healing in this country, and especially among its disadvantaged communities and groups.

In the sixties, as a community health nurse, I was among those who used the tools of the street, of community organizing on the ground, face-to-face work to bring about healthier conditions in neighborhoods where they were most needed. The result was a neighborhood health and child care center that served a densely populated area until Reagan-era budget cuts closed it (see my 1970 book, *9226 Kercheval: The Storefront that Did Not Burn*, published by the University of Michigan Press).

Today, with austere budgets at almost every governmental level and every type of nonprofit service, there can be few professionals or others doing face-to-face street work; nor may they be welcome. The new information technologies can become a new set of tools able to support many new tasks in ways that fit better in today's world. They could help outsiders connect with local, less advantaged communities, and could help communities become advocates and not just recipients of uncertain and diminishing generosity by advantaged Americans.

But much must be done before that can happen. We are very good at establishing oases of innovation. It is the rest of the job, extending the benefits to all who need them, that never seems to get done, often because spreading the good things equitably requires leadership in public policy, and political courage requires public support.

This book attempts to present an in-depth look at some of these homegrown, inventive oases in community information technology and the issues and policy prospects that may or may not bring their benefits to the rest of America.

ACKNOWLEDGMENTS

THE AUTHOR acknowledges with gratitude the partial support for this work by funds and in-kind support from the Kellogg Foundation; the Carrington Faculty Fund, School of Nursing, University of North Carolina at Chapel Hill; NIH Biomedical Research Support Grant #5-343-47; Case Western Reserve College of Nursing, and the College of Health and University of Humberside, U.K.

Special thanks are due, for their personal and professional support, to Dr. Patricia Brennan, Richard Parish, Jean Parthum, and Marie Sullivan, and to all those people in the case study communities and in Washington, D.C., whom I cannot name, who took time and had the patience to talk with me; to them I am most grateful. I also appreciate those who took time to comment on an early draft of the text: Rhonda Galbally, Australia; Irving Rootman, Canada; and Evelyne deLeeuw, The Netherlands.

PART

I

Overview and Introduction

Public health is what we, as a society, do collectively to assure the conditions in which people can be healthy

Institute of Medicine, *The Future of Public Health*, 1988

We all declare for liberty; but in using the same word we do not all mean the same thing. *With some the word liberty may mean for each man to do as he pleases with himself, and the product of his labor; while with others the same may mean for some men to do as they please with other men, and the product of other men's labor. Here are two, not only different, but incompatible things, called by the same name—liberty.*

Abraham Lincoln

They always put highways in low-income neighborhoods; but I ain't seen any of the information highway yet. . . . Why is it easier for my son to get hold of a gun than a computer?

Members of a low-income urban community

CHAPTER

1

AIMS AND MEANS

THIS BOOK is not about computers. It is about ordinary people who are doing new things with computers to create healthier standards and styles of living. They are using these new tools to build social and economic renewal in their communities and to create *community*—the sense of shared responsibility that must accompany and complement viable communities. The stories of community-based information technology (IT) portrayed in the center section of this book focus on experiences of and with economically disadvantaged people whose lives are further burdened by unequal access to education, jobs, housing, and health care because of their race, ethnicity, age, sex, or geographical location. Their stories raise the question of whether these kinds of community-friendly IT ventures will survive as tools to help them do the essential work of building healthier communities. The final chapters search for answers in a critical look at the new policies and policymaking processes that are shaping the national information infrastructure (NII)—the emerging electronic network of networks and information media—in this decade of health care reform.

Competing Visions

Science and Commerce

Today's computers can transmit the contents of the *Encyclopedia Britannica* in three days. In the foreseeable future, the task will take less than one second at a speed of 1 billion bits (one gigabit) per second (one character needs about eight bits of digitized signals). This is the dream of the relatively few users of supercomputers in science, government, and industry. Critics say that such high-performance information technology, with its high expense, is not as important a national goal as expanding the applications of IT to support major societal needs (Huth and Gould 1993; Pagels 1988).

Alternative visions abound. The *commercial* world of telecommunications services and carriers foresees how residents will bank and shop at home, obtain city permits, file federal tax returns, study for college entrance exams, play games, access movies, and traverse foreign places, bodies, and buildings at the flick of a button through interactive IT and "virtual reality," the replication of the world in electronic space (Grossman 1994; Krueger 1990). This vision pictures an unbounded shopping and services mall in the protective surroundings of one's home. Critics say that "profitizing" the electronic world will rule out universal access by making it unaffordable for some groups of Americans.

Employers see the NII as a route to efficiency and flexible organization, saving costs in travel, time, congestion, direct supervision, and personnel. Critics say that the time-bridging, distance-spanning efficiencies of the new information technologies may be at least partially offset by the loss of richer, nuanced person-to-person communications that go on at all meetings and that also seem essential in other nonroutine social and personal affairs (Galegher, Kraut, and Egido 1990).

Public Service, Populism, and the Public Interest

The *public service* view was stated by the vice president as one part of the Clinton administration's vision for the NII:

> The full potential of the National Information Infrastructure will not be realized unless all Americans who desire it have easy, affordable access to advanced communications and information services, regardless of income, disability, or location. . . . It is a goal of this Administration that by the year 2000, all of the classrooms, libraries, hospitals, and clinics in the United States will be connected to the NII. (Gore 1994)

Others would add a *populist* perspective. Through electronic networks people would have a more direct role in making the major political decisions that affect their own lives—more direct democracy and less representative democracy. But critics of populism fear this policymaking by electronic polling could be dominated by a tyranny of the majority, or by the ill-informed, who cannot or do not "consult the rich voice of prior experience . . . outline probable consequences . . . define alternatives . . . or express the nuances of the arguments pro and con" (Grossman 1994).

In contrast to populist, referendum-like decision making, a *public interest* vision would build the capacity of community-based organizations through NII resources to enlarge their role as intermediaries, empowering local people, helping search for information, encouraging dialogue among groups and individuals locally and beyond, assisting moves toward informed agreement on local and national issues, and speaking with and for the interests of those whose voice is little heard.

Form and Framework

These visions and their variants are not mutually exclusive, but in the real world of policy and financing only one or two are likely to shape the NII overall. The worlds that they envision are woven through the discussions and case studies and policy debates presented in this book. The public interest perspective is more thoroughly explored in Part II, the case studies. Part II is preceded in Part I by discussions of reports, research, and viewpoints on the other approaches to information technology. Part III follows up with a focus on policymaking and includes interviews with federal officials in the final part of the book.

This introductory section (Part I) first provides an overview of the entire book (Chapter 2) and then describes the landscape (Chapter 3) through which the NII—the "information superhighway"—is proliferating. One important element of the U.S. expanse, mirrored in the cases, is the widening gap between the most affluent and others—a legacy of the eighties, when the richest fifth of families increased their share to about half of the national income while all others got less, and the poorest fifth of families were left with 4.4 percent of the nation's income (Peterson 1994). Chapter 3 provides a glimpse of the economic, social, and technological scene and is followed by a view of health and the care of health in the context of NII and health care reform policy (Chapter 4).

The second part of the book (Chapters 5–14) portrays five cases in community information technology, each involving different kinds of organizations and communities, populations and purposes, and each preceded by a short review chapter on similar experiences recorded in the literature and recent reports that serve as background to the case studies. Organization requires not only communication, but also coordination, collaboration, leadership, and effective decision making, which can be done, at least in part, on electronic pathways. The case studies in this section demonstrate how.

Each case presents the climate in which the IT venture occurred and the social and economic nature of mainly urban settings and their populations, focusing on disadvantaged groups and communities. The context suggests some of the reasons for particular groups to attempt to use IT, such as budget pressures and growing social needs. The innovations in IT at the grass roots level are traced from the source of the idea in a parent organization to fruition as "facts on the ground," with description and analysis of the hurdles, barriers, assists, and maneuvers that brought them into being and kept them going. Part II closes with a summary (Chapter 14) that brings together the common elements, themes, problems, processes, consequences, and issues for policy attention that the case studies present.

The final part of the book sketches the policy environment in the first half of the nineties, outlining the policy views of the major players in and outside the federal government. Most of the material is based on interviews conducted in key organizational units in the Clinton administration, Congress, and the federal bureaucracy done in the fall of 1993. The book ends with an epilogue on prospects and a proposal for community information technology policy based on the cases and observations of federal agencies in the months following the initial studies in 1993.

Approach

This book focuses on on-site, detailed case studies in community information technology and their policy relevance, which was further developed by extensive interviews with federal policy officials. The *purpose* was to try to understand what kinds of processes and problems organizations in poor communities face in developing their IT capacity, to draw policy implications from these findings, and then to assess the feasibility of policy support for information technology capacity-building in the current federal policy environment. The conceptual *working proposition* used in this work is that a program or policy issue, whether in an organization in a community or in Washington, draws the attention of public and private groups that see a prospective program or policy change as important to their interests. This occurs within a social context that is enabling or restrictive. The groups (stakeholders) use their resources to influence the shape, pace, or direction of change in ways that will enhance or at least not harm their interests. The effectiveness of their efforts depends on their influence, status, resources, and skill compared with competing groups. The interplay among them determines whether and in what form a program or policy moves through various phases from initiation to adoption, implementation, and beyond.

Methods

Case studies are well suited as tools for understanding unexplored areas of social experience such as the use of community information technology. They allow us to obtain information and to derive lessons or "working rules of thumb" (rather than just explaining events or testing a theory). They also, in this instance, serve to help those who are unacquainted with the possibilities of community information technology to envision them in a practical sense. These illustrations are intended to make this material more useful and credible to potential users, whether practitioners, organizations, educators, or policymakers. In addition, they should help focus attention on small-scale community users and uses, to garner support for strengthening their communities and promoting people's well-being and health.

The policy-related component of this work was undertaken to help make the policy implications of the cases relevant to the organizational and political priorities of decision makers. It was an effort to assess the feasibility of policy support for community information technology among relevant federal officials, to take account of their perspectives and the policy environment in which they are working.

The particular case study *sites* were selected for their diversity from a computerized literature search and an earlier pilot study based on a mail survey and on-site interviews, as well as informal, word-of-mouth sources. The site visits and interviews (including the policy study) took place between December 1991 and October 1993. Each lasted from three days to two weeks, depending on the availability of the interviewees and the complexity of the situation.

The *informants* were selected on the basis of the previsit information and through a "snowball" process on advice from informants at the site. The interviewees were members of the stakeholder organizations that affected or were affected by the community IT venture. The individuals were in positions of responsibility and authority in the community information technology program. They could provide contrasting perspectives on events, and could represent the position of their organizational unit as well as their personal opinions. In all there were 77 interviewees in the case studies and 18 interviewees in the policy study.

The *interviews* were semistructured and focused on the initiation, implementation, and maintenance of the IT programs. This included exploration of the processes involved, the problems faced and how they were dealt with (especially resource issues), a description of the IT program itself, and any attempt at evaluating its impact. The informants were also asked their views on the background of the organization, why it became involved with the program, what it hoped to gain, the chronology of events in the history of the IT venture, and expectations about its future. In the policy study, the focus was on current policies in various phases of development, support for the community IT, and whether support was likely or possible in the future.

Informants were assured of strict confidentiality of their person and, in the case studies, of their organization and jurisdiction. Fictitious names are used in the case descriptions below the regional or multistate level. Otherwise, all data—socioeconomic, political, health-related, and institutional—are site-specific and empirical. Quoted and noncited material in the text is drawn mainly from the interviews, and occasionally from written sources that are not cited to avoid identifying the site. Other sources of information were archival data in the form of memos, reports, planning documents, fiscal data, computer printouts, newspaper clippings, and public survey data.

A more detailed description of the framework and methods used for this book is in the Appendix.

References

Galegher, J., R. Kraut, and C. Egido (eds.) 1990. *Intellectual Teamwork: Social and Technological Foundations of Cooperative Work*. Hillsdale, NJ: Lawrence Erlbaum.

Gore, A. 1994. Statement on the National Information Infrastructure Initiation. Washington, DC: The White House, 11 January.

Grossman, L. 1994. "Reflections on Life along the Electronic Superhighway." *Media Studies Journal* 8 (1): 27–40.

Huth, V., and S. Gould. 1993. *The National Information Infrastructure: The Federal Role*. Washington, DC: Library of Congress, November.

Krueger, M. 1990. *Artificial Reality*. New York: Addison-Wesley.

Pagels, H. 1988. *Dreams of Reason. The Computer and the Rise of the Sciences of Complexity*. New York: Simon and Schuster.

Peterson, W. 1994. *Silent Depression: The Fate of the American Dream*. New York: Norton.

CHAPTER

2

THEMES AND ISSUES

THIS OVERVIEW gives a chapter-by-chapter description of the rest of the book, pointing out the highlights of the discussions, case experiences, and conclusions.

Background

The Scene

Chapter 3, "The U.S. Landscape, Information Superhighway, and Electronic Hitchhikers," first sketches the overall national environment in which the new information technologies (IT) are developing, and the rapid growth and economic strength of the industry. It notes the effects of corporate uses of IT in a competitive global economy on a workforce that has growing numbers of women and young people. It compares the access of some Americans to the technologies to their disadvantaged counterparts. And it points out that the policy focus of the Clinton administration and Congress on accelerating the national information infrastructure (NII) will be a very mixed blessing, depending on who sits at the negotiating table and whose interests are served in making the policies that are shaping the NII.

The chapter ends with the caution that throughout NII development, the demands for equity are being confronted by powerful and articulate voices for the free market that would bypass, defer, or let trickle-down the benefits of IT for disadvantaged communities. Such disregard, benign or not, would speed up the widening gap between haves and have-nots. At the heart of the debates is the equity-enterprise pull and tug, a David and Goliath effort.

The stakes go beyond the vast potential for profit in the IT marketplace. The NII will be more than the kind of conduit to information and communication that the old penny press and telephone or television were. The new electronic networks will be tools that can give birth to new organizations and revive old ones, can activate and mobilize groups of people, coalitions, communities for social, health, and economic development, and can be a new and more effective channel for public and political participation beyond the one-way modes of the past and the privileged access of the few. With federal leadership and policy support, the new information technologies could bring a burst of new "soft technologies," new social arrangements that can revive disadvantaged communities, creating the basic conditions for health.

The case portrayals of recent experiences with community information technology—the organized application of IT by and with disadvantaged communities to enable their well-being and health—illustrate the laborious and often tenuous efforts being undertaken with only a patchwork of resources and without the support of public policy. By contrast, support has long been given to large-scale corporate, governmental, and other educational and service organizations.

What Is a Healthy Community?

Chapter 4 weaves the connections between health and its community roots, health care, IT, and public policy. It argues that *health* security is not the same as *health care* security. Health security entails moving away from today's disabled longevity and inequalities in health toward healthy longevity and health equity. These cannot be reached by health care alone.

Both material resources and intergroup cooperation are necessary to ensuring healthy communities. If public health and health care agencies can support local groups in developing local resources—ranging from housing to health care—and work with them, they can promote health. Information technology provides a new set of tools that can be used for these purposes by communities and with communities.

Health requires, according to the classic definition of public health, not only health services but also the "development of social machinery that will ensure to every individual in the community a standard of living adequate for the maintenance of health." Without collective responsibility—as expressed in a health-supporting infrastructure that gives people options in housing, education, jobs, health care, and child care—no individual could "take responsibility for their own health."

In a discussion of *community*, the point is made that a kind of social entropy seems to have accelerated in the last quarter-century, a social and physical distancing of groups of people. To some extent, electronic communication joins people. But electronic communities must be made of like-minded individuals and are not substitutes for local face-to-face communities. Community in *spirit* and in *a place* are two sides of a coin. People who do not feel bound together cannot build together. Without building livable communities, well-being and health are not achievable.

The main theme of the chapter is that the essentials for building healthy communities clearly speak to a complex societal web tied to public policies—fiscal, economic, education, civil rights, labor, environmental, housing, social services, and health care. A new part of this protective and health-supporting infrastructure is the new information technologies. They are a new set of tools to build the "social machinery" that can support health.

The chapter outlines how information technology can favorably impact on people's health in both obvious and more subtle ways. It can provide information on healthy living, on how to access health services, and on how to connect with supportive groups that share common health problems. It can help public and private health services delivery systems be more efficient and effective. But information technology also offers information, referral, and communications links to the broader health-supporting resources that sustain healthy standards of living, such as opportunities for education, job training, child care, and income assistance. Finally, electronic networks support community organizations, improving their services and making them more effective coalition-builders and advocates for better local and national policies and programs.

The prospect of restructured, more integrated health care systems offers a context for using IT in ways that go beyond cost-saving administrative and clinical uses. With IT, health organizations could also join more closely with community-based groups and engage in mutually supportive, collaborative activities to promote health and prevent disease throughout communities.

Delivering Health Services

Each case study in Part II illustrates several of the ways that information technology, usually in the form of computers and computer networks, can affect health. Chapters 6 and 8 present cases that emphasize information, referral, and communication benefits through electronic access to and delivery of health care. Similar information technology benefits from health-supporting resources like education and jobs are highlighted in Chapters 9, 11, and 13. Organization and advocacy through information technology are seen in Chapters 8 and 13, which illustrate the importance of adequate housing and civil rights in a health-supporting community.

Current Uses of IT

As background for the first case study, Chapter 5 reviews recent literature and reports on current uses of IT in the delivery of health services.

Attention has been focused on IT's usefulness to providers and on technical issues rather than on patients, families, or communities and actual community-based services. In the private sector, primary attention has been given to patient record systems and telemedicine—digital radiology, virtual reality simulation of medical procedures, and diagnostic support systems. In public health agencies, access to disease rates, regulations, training materials, and emergency notices have been the focal point of IT use.

Systemwide pressures on health care delivery, including cost constraints and public accountability, mean that new attempts will be made to use IT to improve health care efficiency and effectiveness. Effectiveness and cost control will require reaching underserved groups, satisfying patients, and improving patients' health under new mandates for access and quality.

Although the health care literature on IT remains focused on providers, there is a suggestion of movement toward new areas of interest, from administration to services, from hospital to community, from providers to consumers, from individuals to homes and families and community groups. In some locales, professionals have used IT for delivering some community health services. But these services often have an individual focus, a case management kind of approach. Other communities, envisioning a broader approach, have often failed before they could begin.

Without technical support and basic community resources, IT cannot build communities. Far more than technical and professional issues are involved in any future successes with IT in health services delivery. Soft technology, involving people and organizational relations along with the resources to support time-consuming transitions, is as essential as hard technology. These and other issues revealed in the written record suggest that extensive training and seed monies for communities and other supports will be needed to enable the potential uses of IT in health care delivery to be realized in the foreseeable future.

With both the promise and the precautions suggested by these experiences to provide perspective, the book moves into the first detailed case in community information technology.

Supporting Home Caregivers

"Supporting Home Caregivers in Indy," Chapter 6, portrays the experience of a moderate sized, industrial city with a type of community information technology called CareNet. CareNet was an electronic network connecting patients with Alzheimer's Disease or with AIDS, and their family caregivers, with health professionals and with each other for the duration of their illness. The chapter examines the urban community and organizational environments that provided the incentives and supports, as well as deterrents, for the development and sustainability of the network.

The experience suggests that an innovation, once begun, must be mothered by ongoing organized support, and that the groups using IT—health and social services professionals, organization staff, and patients and families in their homes—need continuing back-up support in the form of retraining, upgrading, and technical troubleshooting.

Supporting Outcasts and Neighborhoods

Reaching Out

Chapter 7, "Reaching Out with Information Technology," discusses reports of how early uses of IT support professional *providers* of educational and social services. The emphasis again is on information transfer, not the exploration of communication and organizational possibilities on behalf of or in conjunction with community groups. Nonetheless, alongside the technology applications, social creations—social or soft technology—if sometimes abortive, are emerging to the benefit of children and elders and community organizations.

To develop IT's potential in childhood education, research suggests that teaching habits will need to move beyond current teacher-centered delivery systems that use computers as knowledge-dispensing machines—like the conventional emphasis in the health care system.

Among the elderly, IT can provide self-support tools for everyday living, such as electronic reminders and instructions for medications. But these may not be used extensively in the foreseeable future. One reason is that IT equity cannot exist as long as poverty remains significant among certain groups of the elderly, especially women. But frail or robust, the elderly are able to learn to use computers to extend their contacts, and are willing to take on some of the tasks that once meant dependence on professionals and others. Chapter 9 demonstrates this point, and early research supports it.

One elder support network failed not only because of hardware problems, but for many more "soft" (organizational) problems: lack of computer consultants, staff attrition, and new staff not having the training to use the computerized system. The social infrastructure was not as developed as the hard technology.

An Electronic Safety Net

Chapter 8, "An Electronic Safety Net in Southcity," shows why information technology does not talk unless people want it to do so. Soft technology must advance far enough to enable hard technology to work. The chapter describes an attempt to build a metropolitan-wide IT network, Clearinghouse for Emergency Aid to the Community (CHEC), in a large, southern city. CHEC contained a shared database of all public and nonprofit services, allowing coordination among agencies, including shared client records.

The story portrays religious and nonprofit groups engaging in bargaining and competition and at times restricting services available to poor and homeless people because of their moral precepts and other interests. Turf warfare, organizational control over client lists, and disagreement over which organizations could be included in the network, what services should be listed in the database, and which clients would be denied services (such as birth control or abortion) illustrate the information and collaboration issues that will arise hundreds of times as community groups attempt to interconnect electronically.

The CHEC episode shows how one of its client organizations, a religious hospital corporation, spun off a variety of structures to address changes in health care policy. It used IT to support and create a new system, discovering workable arrangements to marry IT with present practice and future needs of the community. The St. Francis Health System delivered mobile health services to the poor on the streets of Southcity using laptop IT at 80 sites, tailoring visits to the needs of people at housing shelters, food centers, and churches.

Elders in Action

A second case of reaching out with IT, this time into poor neighborhoods in a small midwestern city, is told in the story of "Elders in Action: Using Information Technology with Young and Old in Midcity" (Chapter 9). Led by retired elders, this community demonstrated that an electronic network needs a social net to give it birth and sustain its berth in community life. The decades old, church-sponsored Friends House wove a set of community IT programs into its community to help children, single mothers, and institution-bound elders change their lives.

Working and Learning at a Distance

Economic Enterprise and Education

Chapter 10 explores the *transfer of work and educational activities instead of people* to accomplish paid work and learning at a distance from employers and teachers. From documented experiences in the United States and other countries, it reveals how the new information technologies are creating new patterns of economic production and new forms of off-site employment, in homes and at local IT centers, to accommodate social as well as economic imperatives. These new forms are becoming bridges between work, education, and home, bringing together information, IT services, and users.

The chapter reviews the major changes in social and employment patterns that are behind these "telecommuting" and "telelearning" ventures, including the corporate effort to gain competitive advantage while accommodating employee family life.

Bringing Business to Hill Park, United Kingdom

Chapter 11 gives a detailed case account of the British brand of IT centers, called "telecottages," and the network of variations that have proliferated throughout the country.

Planners for Hill Park devised the Hill Park Telebusiness Center to provide a local site for business services and offices, job and management training, education and voluntary services support, and home-worker back-up and translation services, all in an attractive and accessible location. The center helped address economic and social problems that are typical of many semirural areas in the United States and Europe—the loss of primary industries, outmigration of young people, and gentrification as "ex-urbanite" professionals build expensive housing to give themselves respite from their high-pressure, high-paying jobs in the cities.

The Hill Park story shows how the initiators of the telebusiness center and their counterparts in other IT centers across England had clear, multipurpose, sometimes altruistic plans for their centers. Yet the centers were shaped by the interests of their many sponsoring groups—local town councils, rural development commissions, job training programs, and especially the telecommunications giant that supported several centers and became a commercial beneficiary. The experiences suggest the need for careful planning so that the interests of external patrons do not distort the direct or indirect health-supporting potential of information technology programs to provide adequate incomes and living conditions.

Responsive Government

IT and Democracy

Chapter 12, "Information Technology and Participatory Democracy," provides background for the final case study on IT as tools for governance. The chapter briefly reviews the connections between earlier forms of information technology and public participation in public decision making, and assesses public issue awareness and activity today on the basis of recent surveys. The significance for health and well-being of effective participation by all social groups, beyond intrinsic social justice, is that without it, policymaking and resource allocation can be inequitable and damaging to the creation of healthy communities.

Active, mainly better-off citizens have their voices heard through their chosen groups, whether a political party, occupational group, profession, union, or interest groups involved in business, church, civil rights, or environmental or social welfare issues. These groups voice members' concerns and preferences, recruit policymakers to their cause, persuade the public and voters, and throughout these activities, collect, develop, and disseminate information. None of these policy-relevant actions could be sustained by individuals acting alone, and all the groups have become more efficient and effective through the use of IT. Individual citizens, in fact, often turn first to citizen groups to help them interpret and use information about public issues. The legal availability of information is not enough to produce effective action.

Giving Voice to the Voiceless

The final case (Chapter 13) portrays a local government in a small, affluent urban community in the southwest that extended its electronic net in ways that enabled citizens to act independently as well as in partnership with their governors. "Giving Voice to the Voiceless in Westsun" is the story of the public information network (PIN) that provided electronic access to city information and services, as well as communication with officials, the public, other individual citizens, and community organizations. One of its aims was to promote a sense of community among its increasingly diverse population. Access was made easier by providing dozens of conveniently placed computers in public places, from libraries to youth centers.

Some PIN users went beyond seeking information and communication, beyond building a sense of "virtual (electronically based) community." They began to create organizations, "virtual organizations," electronic groups that were cohesive enough to have influence and take action in the face-to-face world. One became a formally incorporated organization whose "homed and homeless" members had a significant influence on Westsun's homelessness programs.

The same program, if ventured in poor communities, would have required searching for funds, contacts, expertise, and facilities, and would have been done on volunteer, patchwork time through trial and error, taking much longer and perhaps failing at any juncture along the way.

Some Lessons from the Cases

Making Connections: Common Problems, Processes, and Impacts

The final chapter of Part II (Chapter 14) joins the threads running through the case studies and summarizes the issues related to building IT capacity in community-based organizations in disadvantaged areas. It raises the question of whether the cases represent oddities on the landscape, mere cul-de-sacs linked to the information highway, or a potential force to bring communities that have been socially and economically sidelined into mainstream action.

The chapter first briefly reviews the circumstances and processes that made possible the innovations in community information technology. The way the communities developed community IT, the problems they faced, and the strategies they used to deal with them suggest the kinds of policy support that are needed to make them more than cul-de-sacs, to have them become portraits of the potential for a new set of IT tools to develop health-supporting communities.

The general public and the specific publics that each community focused on obtained a wide range of information, became computer literate, and got basic services such as medical and nursing advice, translation services, library books, and referral services. But the services used most often on the network were intergroup and individual communication rather than information. Community IT became more than a way to deliver health, social, educational, and business information and services at relatively little cost. It became a resource for organizational renewal and for new organization development.

The IT possibilities in this book are not viewed as a perfect or complete solution to the issues involved in improving the health and quality of life of disadvantaged groups. Rather, they represent a new set of tools, which if effectively shared, will allow people to derive IT's potential benefits and help less advantaged communities avoid falling further behind in community development, health, and life.

Making Policy

Part III addresses the policy implications of the case studies based on interviews with officials in Washington, D.C., and on subsequent observations by the author. "The Information Technology Policy Environment" (Chapter 15) outlines the policies that emerged in the 1990s with the new political agenda in technology and health care reform. Following a brief discussion of changes in the old media and the increasing mismatch between federal regulation and emerging electronic media, the major issues that are shaping the National Information Infrastructure are laid out. These are followed by the positions of the major stakeholders in government, business, education, and the nonprofit services and public interest communities.

A variety of congressional bills introduced in the mid-1990s ensured that all major constituencies, ranging from the general public to large businesses and nonprofit institutions, would be supported with special resources to enter and help create the electronic future on the NII. All constituencies were included, except for the small-scale, low-budget, community-based organizations in disadvantaged areas.

Policy Prospects for Community Information Technology

Chapter 16 is an epilogue offering a view of policy prospects for community information technology, including suggestions for policy support derived from the case studies and the policy environment. Virtually all responsible federal agencies and interest groups, when faced with the question of how out-of-the-mainstream organizations that are too poor to develop an information technology capacity would become part of the National Information Infrastructure, said they had given the issue little, if any, attention.

Community institutions often form bridges between residents and outside, large-scale government, corporate, and other organizations led by professionals. Left to the vagaries of the market, these organizations may find their attempts to develop IT programs shaped by the vision of an electronic shopping mall rather than as tools to build healthy communities. They require a share of the public funds for information technology development.

To remedy the extensive information technology deficits in organizations in poor communities, the remaining pages of the book describe the concept of community IT support centers, to be seeded by federal funds. These centers would be counterparts to those becoming available in more favored communities for schools, libraries, businesses, or as freestanding entities.

Under the control of a local coalition of organizations, these first-stop, one-stop centers could provide a range of services to small local organizations, including technology transfer and liaison, public education, convening of interested parties, and brokering organizational relationships to acquire needed resources. They would be catalysts for IT development.

By including the creation of such enabling systems for small-scale organizations in the vision of an electronic future, an IT infrastructure would be built at the grass roots, offering more fertile ground for healthier, cohesive communities.

CHAPTER

3

THE U.S. LANDSCAPE, INFORMATION SUPERHIGHWAY, AND ELECTRONIC HITCHHIKERS

How the Wonders of Information Technology Are Not All Blessings

POSTING HIS message—the "95 Theses"—on an Augsburg church door in 1520, the priest Martin Luther began a revolution, the Protestant Reformation, which asserted the right of men and women to communicate directly with their God.

Today, Lutherans can post messages across the country to each other as individuals or collectively through LUTHERLINK. They are joined by Jews on JEWISHNET and Mennonites on MENNOLINK, along with dozens of other religious groups, who can also communicate with each other on other parts of ECUNET, the ecumenical electronic network that offers computer bulletin boards, conferencing, and other services to its subscribers on a nonprofit basis (Lee 1991). Users gain access with a modem, attaching their computer to their telephone line and dialing up the network.

Tomorrow electronic networks will be able to host interconnections and other communications and information services among virtually every group of users any time, anywhere in the world. How fast this will occur and how universal it will be—which groups will be left on the roadbed of the "information superhighway" begging to hitch a ride—will depend on the vision and foresight of policymakers and the organized voices that speak for the interests of the public, including less visible, disadvantaged communities.

At its outset, Clinton administration policy called for acceleration of the national information infrastructure (NII)—the networking of electronic networks (encompassing all forms of transmission: optical fiber or telephonic twisted copper wiring, wireless satellite, line-of-sight microwave, and broadcast) and information media (television, computers, compact disks, publishing, video) (Clinton 1993). This is to be the new lifeline to information, communication, enterprise, and services—to participation, organization, and community. Its major shapers, alongside government, are the network owners, the appliance (computers, television, telephone) and information providers, and the customers and users—businesses, educational and other public institutions, the general public, and the low-budget community organizations that are often closest to the people whose voice is least heard in the policy forums. All of these players have a clear interest in the unfolding reality of the NII.

If the voiceless are heard during the next decade of NII design, not only will they gain access to the benefits of the network as recipients, but they could also become providers of information, ideas, services, development. In so doing, they could potentially become more socially cohesive, stronger "communities of interest," and more health-supporting "communities of place."

The technological advances of the telematics revolution are stunning. The social "soft technologies"—the arrangements that determine their use, by and for whom, when, and at what cost—are much less advanced by comparison.

A Glimpse of the Information Technology Industry

Information technology (IT) transmits and represents information (facts, data, or opinions in any format, textual, numerical, graphic, or audiovisual) and creates the hardware and software that processes it (OMB 1993). The technologies that will make up the NII are part of a vast and rapidly growing information technology industry, responsible for 12 percent of the nation's gross domestic product and comparable to the trillion-dollar health care industry (Gore 1993a). In 1991, U.S. capital spending on computers and communications equipment was greater than capital investment in traditional industrial equipment (Stewart 1994).

Semiconductors, the microchips at the heart of computerized systems, were worth $61 billion worldwide in the early nineties. The microchip of the mid-nineties, at 0.004 the diameter of a strand of hair, could store the information of a 200-volume encyclopedia. Personal computers (PCs), first introduced for practical purposes in 1981, grew to $93 billion in sales in ten years, and software revenues, growing at 25 percent a year, amounted to $125 billion around the world in 1990 (Kelly 1991; Finklestein 1992).

Computers and their linkages to telecommunications are now embedded in much of the U.S. economy. Almost every job in the future will be affected by these technologies. More than half of all jobs were information based by the early 1990s; more than four in ten business people used computers to access 39,000 commercial databases in the

United States, compared to fewer than one in ten workers using 900 databases in Japan ("Technology Payoff" 1993; Kelly 1991; Pollack 1993).

New Technologies

Just as the advances in information technology in organized work places had built on previous tools, from pen and ink to standardized file boxes and forms, the technological advances of the early nineties built on the spread of hardware and software of the previous decade (Yates 1989). Multimedia capacity became increasingly common, allowing interactive use of computers that could support sound, still images, animation, or full-motion video (Strothman 1991). Compact optical disks (CDs) for computers with CD drives contained up to 285,000 pages of machine readable text (CD-ROM with 600MB of data), including geological surveys, census information, financial market data, and reference books. They became available free of charge from some government sources, but could also cost up to several hundred or thousands of dollars from commercial sources (GAO 1992b).

Business users could engage in real-time video conferencing with the option of sharing screens and transferring files between users through their desktop computers, making possible collaborative work, meetings, and presentations regardless of physical distance (Papp 1993).

Telephone companies upgraded their pairs of electricity-carrying copper wires to fiber-optic cable—hair-thin glass wires that use pulses of light (laser beams)—to transmit hundreds of television channels, telephone calls, and computer data. Fiber optics can carry 30,000 times the conversations of traditional lines, and do so more quickly, clearly, and cheaply (OTA 1991). The market for these proliferating webs more than doubled in the last decade (Stewart 1994).

In remote areas, where the cost of providing wireline service is prohibitive, wireless services—line-of-sight microwave, radio, and satellite technologies—became available. In these and other communities where fiber-optic cables were not yet installed, the building blocks of an enlarging network—local, wide, and metropolitan area networks (LANs, WANs, and MANs)—proliferated. LANs are relatively limited in their reach, usually covering the premises of a building or a campus, or related businesses. More than half of all PCs were connected by over 5 million LANs in the early 1990s, allowing people with similar interests to find each other. And like the telephone, they tend to reinforce community ties (OTA 1991).

Regional networks were among the more than 8,500 U.S. and foreign networks linked to the "backbone" Internet, which forms the base electronic network across the country and is to become the trunk along which the NII will proliferate. The Internet is anchored by FIXs (Federal Internet Exchanges) and was managed by NASA, the U.S. Department of Energy, and the National Science Foundation to provide remote access to their supercomputers. The overall management of the Internet was in the hands of a coalition of universities (OTA 1993a).

New Work Organization

These technologies also allowed companies to "reengineer" the ways they produce goods and services, and began to create new patterns of work and employment. After businesses spent a trillion dollars on IT in the 1980s, productivity rose faster than economic growth in the 1990s. A half-million clerical and technical staff were no longer needed and were replaced by 120,000 new software personnel ("Technology Payoff" 1993). These job losses especially affected women, who make up about 80 percent of clerical workers but fewer than 30 percent of programmers and systems analysts in the United States (Kling and Dunlop 1993). The absolute number of secretaries dropped by 12 percent from a peak of over 4 million in 1988 (Stewart 1994).

Information technology made possible the globalization of commerce, the "virtual corporation"—electronic coordination of production, sales, and financing, whether in another town or a distant hemisphere. This new-style organization could focus on "core competencies" from a "core staff," more short-term and part-time "contingent workers," such as consultants, independent contractors, clerks, and health care staff, as its market grew and shrank with the economy. This led to a net loss of jobs (Brecher 1993; "Technology Payoff" 1993).

Competition, Jobs, and Social Spin-Offs

The IT industry also mirrored other facets of the overall economy, including the loss of market share. Almost 60 percent of the world microchip market was held by U.S. firms in 1980, and almost all computers bought in this country were made here. Ten years later the U.S. world market share for chips dropped by half, and only two-thirds of the U.S. computer market was made up of products made here, again affecting the number, quality, and security of jobs (Kelly 1991).

By the nineties, the labor market became very different from the past. Unemployed people were without jobs for longer periods of time, and only 15 percent (as compared with 44 percent in the past) could expect to return to their former jobs. Many industries reduced their workforce, and in the global competition for markets, they transferred some jobs to other countries. Improved technology eliminated other jobs, and many new jobs were part-time and temporary, paying low wages with few or no benefits (GAO 1993b). As a result, real, inflation-adjusted wages did not grow, nor did the rate of new jobs, and unemployment persisted. This burdened families, especially single parents, and communities, especially the already disadvantaged, and public budgets, especially those already threatened by deficits ("Technology Payoff" 1993; Kelly 1991).

Although advances in technology were thought to be part of the formula for economic recovery, other parts of the solution were infrastructure development and education and training of the workforce. Private and public investment in this support structure had declined to a social and political breaking point by the 1992 U.S. national election (GAO 1993a; Secretary's Commission 1991). A changing job market could not absorb the numbers of unskilled job seekers, who were emerging without diplomas from problem-ridden public schools. Gaps between rich and poor continued to widen throughout the eighties and beyond. Affordable rental housing was available for only half the families who needed it, and affordable health care was beyond reach for over 37 million Americans (Kelly 1991; GAO 1992d, 1992a; Milio 1993; Blendon and Edwards 1991). The widening wage gap between high- and low-paid workers—which had accelerated twice as fast as in Germany or Japan after 1980—made good education less affordable, adding to the education gap and producing an overall decline in the growth of the skilled labor force at a time when the need for skills continued to grow (Bernstein 1994).

New Options

The increasing surplus of freed-up labor time, often viewed as a crisis, could, in the eyes of some analysts, offer a challenge to use human resources for alternative necessary tasks supported by the technologies that minimize painful toil. There is no shortage of work to be done to strengthen community and communities, but much of it is either not highly profitable or not "digitizable" in the ways that manufacturing, finance, entertainment, and science are because they rely on numerical databases. For example, there is work to renew and construct affordable housing and transportation tailored to environmental and personal protection. There are jobs to be done to promote energy conservation and renewable resources; to biomanage agriculture and local produce; to secure safe and attractive neighborhoods, improve schools and libraries, care for the aged and homebound and children; and to encourage and demonstrate shared responsibility for addressing public issues (GAO 1993a).

This work calls for shaping technology and infrastructure to local situations. It takes collaboration and creativity to reinvent IT from a set of mainly information and communications tools for use as organizing, development, and mobilizing tools, activities that are difficult to undertake and sustain but are crucial to creating healthy communities.

Access to Information Technology

Almost all Americans have telephones and televisions. Almost a third had computers in the early 1990s (Stewart 1994). They used them for household management in about three out of four homes, and for education purposes in two out of three homes. Almost half used their computer for work brought home. And almost all these homes also had VCRs (Strothman 1991). A majority of households (60 percent) subscribed to cable television networks, while relatively few (1.2 million, including 4 percent of homes) computers were connected to the Internet and could reach around the world (Pollack 1993; Tierney 1993). About half of American children used a computer at home or at school. Almost every school had at least one computer for instructional use, and 1,000 high schools were connected to the Internet (OTA 1992).

All this made Americans the most networked people in the world, while just 39,000 Japanese were connected to the Internet, and less than 3 in 100 Japanese households were connected to cable television. In the European Union, 1 in 6 homes were linked to cable or satellite television (Pollack 1993; Carat TV 1992).

Commercial Hopes

According to 1993 customer research, Americans subscribed to private computer networks not as a source of information but to communicate with other subscribers; on-line subscribers tripled between 1989 and 1993 (Stewart 1994). Commercial computer networks anticipated interactive TV, a kind of family-friendly form of computer networking, as a new opportunity for innovative advertising—for example, using "virtual reality" to allow viewers to walk through a car or read the details of an insurance policy. Public opinion polls showed that over 90 percent of adults wanted interactive TV and would pay up to $10 more a month for added services. Younger people were even more interested than older ones (Tierney 1993).

This networked TV medium, as used in Montreal, hinted at typical early habits. With interactive video, people added two hours to their TV terminal viewing time, for a total of 8.5 hours a week (4 on video games, 3 on interactive quiz-type TV programs, and the rest on data services such as weather, horoscopes, and lottery numbers (Tierney 1993).

Equity

Whatever the benefits of IT, the tools are not equally shared. Only one in ten people who had less than a high school education used a computer at work or had one at home, compared with two out of three people with postgraduate education. Similarly, four to five times as many people with more than $50,000 annual income used computers at work or home as did poor persons (OTA 1993c; Murdock and Golding 1989). Younger people were at least twice as likely as their elders to use them (Alliance for Public Technology 1990; OTA 1984). Rural and other isolated communities were also often sidelined on the information highway (OTA 1990, 1991), as were schools in poor communities (OTA 1988) and small-scale, community-based organizations, especially those in low-income neighborhoods (Smith 1988; Rubinyi 1989; Rodberg 1991). These were also the groups, organizations, and communities where unemployment and job development, lack of training, education, and infrastructure were most pressing.

Shifts in the Federal Agenda

Viewing IT as a major ingredient to lead as well as support economic growth, trade, education, health care, and government efficiency and effectiveness, the new presidential administration in 1993 shifted away from previous federal priorities and policy initiatives. The traditional approach to communications and information policy had been federal regulation of separate industries, Defense Department–based research and development of computers and communications, and in the eighties, the view that information was a commodity like any other, whether governmentally or privately produced, and so salable at a profit (Dutton, Blumler, and Kraemer 1987).

The policy agenda for the previous 20 years focused on hardware and the commercial implications of IT, such as the changes in the telecommunications industry resulting from AT&T divestiture, deregulation, and the impact of IT on business, commerce, global and domestic stock markets, and financial and health services. Other foci were wireless technologies (cellular phones and personal communications devices), the role of supercomputers, computing technologies for economic competitiveness, and protection of intellectual property rights. Some attention was given to the impact of IT on rural areas, the disabled, office work, and education

(OTA 1993b). The central issues, however, involved large-scale technologies and the interests of large-scale institutions, those of national military security and commercial enterprise. Never was community-based IT on the agenda as an item for debate or support.

The 1990s shifts in priorities and approach to IT policy led to reallocation of a large and increasing share of IT development funds from defense to the Department of Commerce. The use of IT to help reinvent government gained visibility and concerted action (Gore 1993b; Committee on Science 1993; White House 1993a). Information, for policy purposes, became redefined as "a valuable national resource" to ensure accountability, manage government operations, maintain the healthy performance of the economy, and, while it is also a commodity in the marketplace, the "free flow between government and the public is essential to democratic society" (OMB 1993).

Market and Moral Modeling

Because the federal government is the largest single producer, collector, consumer, and disseminator of information in the United States and the world, its activity in information and related technologies shapes markets and affects the practices of lesser institutions, quite apart from the public policies that directly affect them. Mistakes come at a high public cost. For example, when the National Institutes of Health did not effectively manage key aspects of a major information system contract, the result was a cost overrun of $800 million (GAO 1992a). But other practices can have public benefits in the market and serve as a model to emulate.

Beginning in 1993, the government's $20 billion annual budget for technology purchases was to be spent on equipment tagged with the Environmental Protection Agency star, indicating energy-conserving, nonpolluting computers (White House 1993b). These sales would stimulate development and sales of environmentally friendly equipment and widen access for other public and private buyers. Federal attention to the IT capacity of small-scale organizations could have similar large-scale effects.

Information technology was also to be used to support another major policy initiative of the administration—health care reform—with the intention of increasing access to services and lowering costs. Estimates showed that a net savings of up to $5 billion annually in administrative costs could be achieved through creation of a national uniform electronic data transmission format, and that an additional $18 billion could be gained in clinical efficiency from integrated medical data systems (Fuchs and Merlis 1993; Lewin-VHI 1993). Enactment of such a program would not simply model, but would transform health services practices at every level, making possible organizational linkages that might otherwise take years to develop, lowering the costs to health facilities and governments, and stimulating the IT market and related jobs in organizations and communities equipped with the infrastructure to do the job.

An Open Platform?

The policy work for the next decade—the political processes of influence, negotiation, and compromise, and the selection of groups to sit at the table and voice their interests—will determine how real are the democratic ideals of ready access to open information and many-sided communication to ensure public accountability. These ideals, alongside the economic goals outlined in the administration's NII Agenda for Action, reveal the tug of war between the marketplace of ideas and the commercial market in creating the information highway. This tension rings with a cautionary message to attend to the equitable "public right of way" for the general public and for disadvantaged groups, organizations, communities—to allow them to join the shapers of the new directions that IT takes, rather than be relegated as in the past to the status of hitchhikers.

References

Alliance for Public Technology. 1990. "Survey of PC Users." Washington, DC: APT.

Berstein, A. 1994. "Inequality: How the Gap Between Rich and Poor Hurts the Economy." *Business Week*, 15 August, 78–83.

Blendon, R. J., and J. N. Edwards. 1991. "Caring for the Uninsured: Choices for Reform." *Journal of the American Medical Association* 265 (19): 2563–65.

Brecher, J. 1993. *Global Visions: Beyond the New World Order*. Detroit, MI: South End Press.

Carat TV. 1992. "Cable and Satellite Television in Europe." *Eureka* 16: 9.

Clinton, W. 1993. "Technology for America's Economic Growth: A New Direction to Build Economic Strength." Washington, DC: The White House, 22 February.

Committee on Science, Space, and Technology. 1993. *National Information Infrastructure Act of 1993*. Washington, DC, U.S. Congress.

Dutton, W. H., J. G. Blumler, and K. L. Kraemer. 1987. In *Wired Cities: Shaping the Future of Communications*, edited by W. H. Dutton, J. G. Blumer, and K. L. Kraemer. Boston: G. K. Hall.

Finkelstein, J. 1992. *The American Economy. From the Great Crash to the Third Industrial Revolution*. Arlington Heights, IL: Harland Davidson.

Fuchs, B., and M. Merlis. 1993. *Health Care Reform: President Clinton's Health Security Act*. Washington, DC: Congressional Research Service.

General Accounting Office (GAO). 1992a. *Housing Issues*. Washington, DC: U.S. Congress, December.

———. 1992b. *Information Dissemination: Innovative Ways Agencies Are Using Technology*. Testimony before the Government Information, Justice, and Agriculture Subcommittee. Committee on Government Operations, House of Representatives. Washington, DC: U.S. Congress, 19 February.

———. 1992c. *Information Management and Technology Issues*. Washington, DC: U.S. Congress.

———. 1992d. *Poverty Trends, 1980–88: Changes in Family Composition and Income Sources among the Poor*. Testimony before the Subcommittee on Human Resources, Committee on Ways and Means, House of Representatives. Washington, DC: U.S. Congress, 10 September.

———. 1993a. *Choosing Public Investments*. Washington, DC: U.S. Congress, July.

———. 1993b. *Decline in UI Benefits*. Washington, DC: U.S. Congress, September.

Gore, A. 1993a. Address before the National Press Club. Washington, DC. 21 December.

———. 1993b. "From Red Tape to Results: Creating a Government That Works Better and Costs Less." Report of the National Performance Review. Washington, DC: The White House, 7 September.

Kelly, M. 1991. "Preparing for Tomorrow Today." Unpublished paper. Georgia Institute of Technology, Atlanta.

Kling, R., and C. Dunlop. 1993. "Controversies about Computerization and the Character of White Collar Worklife." *Informatics Society* 9: 1–29.

Lee, S. 1991. *Ecunet*. Louisville, KY: Presbyterian Church USA.

Lewin-VHI. 1993. *Reducing Administrative Costs in a Pluralistic Delivery System Through Automation*. Washington, DC: Healthcare Financial Management Association.

Milio, N. 1993. "Approaches to National Health Insurance." In *Nursing Issues in the 1990's*, edited by O. Strickland and D. Fishman. Albany, NY: Delmar.

Murdock, G., and P. Golding. 1989. "Information, Poverty and Political Inequality: Citizenship in the Age of Privatized Communications." *Journal of Communications* 39: 180–85.

Office of Management and Budget (OMB). 1993. *Management of Federal Information Resources.* OMB Circ. A-130. Washington, DC: The White House, 25 June.

Office of Technology Assessment (OTA). 1984. *Technology and Aging in America*. Washington, DC: U.S. Congress.

———. 1988. *Power On! New Tools for Teaching and Learning*. Washington, DC: U.S. Congress, September.

———. 1990. *Critical Connections*. Washington, DC: U.S. Congress, January.

———. 1991. *Rural America at the Crossroads: Networks for the Future*. Washington, DC: U.S. Congress, April.

———. 1992. *Finding a Balance: Computer Software, Intellectual Property, and the Challenge of Technological Change*. Washington, DC: U.S. Congress, April.

———. 1993a. *Advanced Network Technology*. Washington, DC: U.S. Congress, June.

———. 1993b. *Annual Report to the Congress*. Washington, DC: U.S. Congress.

———. 1993c. *Making Government Work: Electronic Delivery of Government Services*. Washington, DC: U.S. Congress, September.

Papp, B. 1993. "Desktop Video-Conferencing System Enters the Multimedia Market." *Telesis*: 81.

Pollack, A. 1993. "Now It's Japan's Turn to Play Catch Up." *New York Times*, 22 November, F1.

Rodberg, L. 1991. "Breaking from Big Brother: Computerizing Small, Government-Funded Organizations." *Computers in Human Services* 8 (1): 105–18.

Rubinyi, R. 1989. "Computer and Community: The Organizational Impact." *Journal of Communication* 39 (3): 110–23.

Secretary's Commission on Achieving Necessary Skills. 1991. *What Work Requires of Schools*. Washington, DC: U.S. Department of Labor.

Smith, L. 1988. "The Development of Computer Applications by Non-Employed People in Community Settings." *Journal of Occupational Psychology* 61 (1): 89–102.

Stewart, T. 1994. "Information Technology." *Fortune*, 4 April, 74–79.

Strothman, J. E. 1991. "Interactive Multimedia: Promise and Pitfalls." Paper presented at the COMDEX O.P.E.N. Conference, Bethesda, MD.

"Technology Payoff." 1993. *Business Week* 14 June, 57–79.

Tierney, J. 1993. "Will They Sit by the TV Set or Ride the Data Highway?" *New York Times*, 20 June, 1, 12.

White House. 1993a. Executive Order. United States Advisory Council on the National Information Infrastructure. Washington, DC, 15 September.

———. 1993b. "Gore Joins Industry Leaders to Unveil Energy-Efficient Computers." White House Press Release. Washington, DC, 17 June.

Yates, J. 1989. *Control Through Communication: The Rise of System in American Management*. Baltimore, MD: Johns Hopkins University Press.

CHAPTER

4

LINKING HEALTH, COMMUNITIES, INFORMATION TECHNOLOGY, AND POLICY

HEALTH SECURITY is not the same as *health care* security. Americans' health assurance lies in addressing twin problems that are undramatic and invisible, but are basic to controlling social costs and health care costs. These problems are disabled longevity from preventable diseases and inequalities in health between better-off Americans and disadvantaged groups, such as low-income persons, African Americans, and Hispanics (Milio 1991). The premise of this book is that the basis for health lies in communities where essential resources are available and where the sense of social cohesion—the other face of "community"—can bring about sufficient distribution of these resources to support health (IOM 1988; Marmot and McDonnell 1986; Kottke 1986). Both material resources and intergroup communication are necessary to ensuring healthy communities. To the extent that health personnel can support local groups in developing resources—ranging from housing to health care—and in working together, they are promoting health. Information technology offers a new set of tools that can be used for these purposes by communities and with communities.

Health Problems

The American population is aging. But it is a disabled, not a healthy longevity. Growing old need not mean being disabled, at least not until those years, beginning around age 85, when human biological potential expires. Most disability is the result of previous decades of illness, mainly chronic physical and mental illness, injury, and birth-related damage. Most health risks originate in human environments—the complex physical, social, economic, and political webs, the ecological nets that can keep people safe through their biological unfolding but can also pose damaging hazards (Kaplan and Camacho 1983; Rosenfeld 1978; Olshansky et al. 1991).

The strategies for health that the nation has used so far have granted longer life, but life with fewer years free from disability than two decades ago. Americans have, in effect, lost two to three disability-free years for every year that has been added to life-expectancy (McKinlay, McKinlay, and Beaglehole 1989; Olshansky et al. 1991). And, although death rates for people over 65 years have improved, the risk of dying in the younger decades, from youth to middle age (the prime years of life), is higher than in other affluent countries (OTA 1993c). The one in five people who make it to old age without disability limitations are able to contribute most to society; they need less than $1,000 in medical care annually (Roos and Havens 1991), compared with the average $2500 or more that elders need.

The burden of disability falls heaviest on the groups that are already disadvantaged by their social and economic condition, which itself declined following cutbacks in public support for several years (GAO 1992d, 1992g). The health of poor children, especially poor black children, declined over the last 15 years (Montgomery 1992). And the official poverty level that determines eligibility for supportive government programs is set too low to sustain average mortality (Keeney 1980).

The Mushrooming Burden

Many years of accumulated evidence show that when risks to health are combined, the damaging effects mushroom in already disadvantaged groups (Williams 1990; Gunning-Schepers 1991). The chances of more illness, more severe forms of illness, more disability, and death are greater among the economically disadvantaged than among others of comparable ages and gender. The earlier in life people incur health deficits, the more risky their future health becomes (Jones 1956; Rice and LaPlante 1986; Kottke 1986; Verbrugge 1985).

Babies with low birthweights, for example, are likely to have more childhood illnesses, impairing their educational achievement and so leading to poorer jobs and lower incomes than they might otherwise have (Williams 1990). People with low incomes face higher risks of life-threatening acute and chronic disease, of disabling diseases, injuries, and death, and of shortened life-expectancy (GAO 1992a; Montgomery 1992; Rogers 1992). They often get inadequate medical care and fewer preventive services, such as public health vaccines, especially if they are black (Steckel 1989; Hutchins et al. 1993). In addition to causing economic hardship, race discrimination impairs doctor-patient relations (Escarce et al. 1993), clinic and cancer care (Lieu, Newacheck, and McManus 1993; Howard et al. 1992), and other types of treatment (Cowie et al. 1993; Hogue and Hargraves 1993). When economically disadvantaged people receive care, they recover less fully and less quickly (OTA 1992a; Oswald 1988; Suzman 1988; Muller 1992). Although the health of economically disadvantaged groups has improved over the decades, it has done so less rapidly than for more advantaged people. The health gap widened, especially during the last decade (Rogers 1992; Montgomery 1992). The mushrooming effects of inequalities of opportunity in education, jobs, and housing produce poverty and its associated high health risks to people who then face further threat when, as members of certain racial and ethnic minorities, they are confronted by limited access to health care and additional discrimination (Milio 1985; Rogers 1992).

Sustainable Health

Movement toward the goals of healthy longevity and health equity—comparable health for all social groups—would mean movement toward sustainable health. That is health security. Sustainable health does not mean living forever. It does mean longevity free from disability caused by avoidable disease and injury. It does not mean patching up, through even a reformed health care system, the damage done to people by unhealthy living and working conditions and environments. It means nurturing a healthy aging people who can use the wealth of their experience in their later decades to work with new generations.

Deficits in Health-Supporting Infrastructure

The nation is not yet on a trajectory for sustainable health, primarily because of many deficits in Americans' health-supporting infrastructure. These deficits can be remedied. The need to rebuild this infrastructure is clear in the following litany of deficits.

Economy, Jobs, and Income

Economic recession, inflation, and unemployment reshape people's lives and underpin much illness (Merva and Fowles 1992; Rogers 1992). The historic record and recent studies known to Congress for almost twenty years show that disease, premature death, and violent death increase when people experience economic desperation and decline in their living conditions (Steckel 1989; Wescott et al. 1985; Smith 1987; Joint Economic Committee 1984). In the past decade, for example, for every 1 percent increase in unemployment, there was more than a 3 to 6 percent increase in deaths from heart disease, stroke, and homicide (Merva and Fowles 1992; Catalano 1991). The health risks caused by added economic strains like job loss are even greater among the already economically disadvantaged (Smith 1987; Wescott et al. 1984; OTA 1986).

Job loss, even in the short term, also means that people defer medical care because of lost income and loss of health insurance. Over the last decade, for every 1 million people who became unemployed, there was a drop of 50,000 hospital admissions (Muller 1992).

Women and Children

An economically secure future is a dim prospect from birth for many who are born into poor households. Not all pregnant women who are eligible for women-infant food benefits have access to them, although these benefits can reduce low-weight births by 25 percent and are cost-effective (GAO 1992a). The national cost of low-weight births—the biggest single hazard to infants—is up to $7 billion annually, and includes birth care that costs $19,000 compared with $3,500 for a normal-weight baby (American Dietetic Assn. 1993). Poor children have the least access to preschool programs. Five million children are ill-prepared to begin school because of poverty-related nutritional, health, and language problems. Retarded growth from undernutrition affects as many as one in seven preschoolers in some low-income groups (GAO 1992f).

Young People

The economic prospects for a third of those in their teens and early twenties and almost 40 million low-income workers declined over the 1980s and early 1990s, which reduced the range of choices for where they could live and work and what they could hope and plan for. At a time when technological change requires new workplace capacities like continued learning, teamwork, managerial skills, and problem solving, they did not have the necessary entry-level skills or access to job training (GAO 1992b).

Yet less than 30 percent of unemployed people received jobless insurance benefits in the early 1990s compared with more than half in the 1950s, and budget-tightening restrictions on unemployment insurance pushed over a quarter million people into poverty in 1990 (GAO 1992b, 1993a). At the same time, the United States jailed ten times more people than the Netherlands and four times as many blacks as apartheid South Africa, and added new jails at heavy financial and social costs (Kennedy 1993).

Having to live on a low income constricts people's lives. Low incomes limit the quality and size of housing, the safety of neighborhoods and choice of workplace, the options for food, fuel, education, stress-free time, and preventive and curative health care, the chances of living in a pollution-free community, and the chances of being heard by policymakers (Milio 1986; Rogers 1992).

The Physical Environment

Another facet of the infrastructure underlying Americans' health is the deterioration of what could once be called the natural environment—air, water, biotic support, and waste control—but which has long been reshaped by government and industry policies. Here too, greater losses and larger health burdens fall on low-income communities where environmental issues such as lead poisoning and incineration have been neglected (Sale 1993). Three to four million preschoolers in the United States have blood lead levels high enough to cause permanent psychological and nervous system impairment (Landrigan 1992).

By the early nineties, the bill to make human habitats humane ballooned: national spending needed to meet environmental goals was $160 billion annually and long-term clean-up of the national defense and energy department installations amounted to $200 billion. Yet, environmental protection operating funds were roughly the same in 1992 as in 1979 (GAO 1992c).

Dwelling Spaces

The dwelling spaces for many working people and neighborhood residents, especially those with low incomes, were often no more safe, secure, or health-supporting than many community habitats. By the early 1990s, there were about 1.7 million disabling workplace injuries, over 350,000 cases of occupational diseases, over 100,000 deaths, and one inspector to monitor the health and safety programs for every 3,000 worksites (GAO 1992f).

The supply of public housing required $20 billion for major repairs, and federal housing had up to $16 billion worth of lead-based paint yet to be removed. At the same time, the private housing market supplied less affordable low-income housing as the need continued to grow: half of low-income families would not be able to find affordable rental housing in the 1990s (GAO 1992d). In order to afford rental housing, families needed a monthly income of about $2,000 or a $13 hourly wage—three times the actual minimum wage (GAO 1993c).

The grim irony here is that federal housing and other investment was being displaced in the federal budget over the eighties and early nineties by the relentless growth of health care costs (GAO 1992e). The high cost of illness was preventing investment in people and places that could prevent much of that illness.

Community, U.S.A.

A kind of social entropy seemed to accelerate in the last quarter of the twentieth century, a social and physical distancing of people. The prime movers of this trend were the growing gap between high-level white-collar occupations and blue-collar production-line workers in declining industries and service jobs. Public policy favored the affluent. More women and young people entered low-paying jobs. Rising divorce rates and more single-person and single-parent households made meeting household budgets and social obligations more difficult (GAO 1993a).

Populations, especially the more affluent and maturing baby boom generation, moved into the interspaces between towns, suburbs, and cities. They, and those following them, have favored privatization of government services, isolation of "our kind," fiscal conservatism, individual rights, and environmental protection as long as their economic interests were not harmed (Louv 1985). These groups were also first to use the new information technologies to multiply occupational contacts, perform professional services, engage in financial transactions, and be informed and entertained (Meyerowitz 1985). Through electronic communications, they discovered "communities of interest," "imagined communities," while acquiring a narrower sense of place and social and local responsibility (Calhoun 1989).

Meanwhile, many job seekers were forced to move to find work, became vulnerable to family break-ups and moved into neighborhoods of increasing violence and deteriorating physical conditions. Social ties to family, workplace, and neighborhood groups were frayed, strained by the loss of income, inadequate public services, and withdrawal of public and private investment (Joint Economic Committee 1984; Catalano 1993; Brenner and Mooney 1983).

Meanings of Community

Electronic communities are not substitutes for local face-to-face communities. Community in spirit and in *a place* are two sides of a coin. People who do not feel bound together cannot build together. Without building livable communities, health and well-being are not achievable.

As the ground for well-being and health, "community" must mean more than detached groups who share communities of interest. Community must also be tied to place, the sense of social responsibility for creating healthy surroundings. This precondition makes other forms of community possible, whether by electronics or with neighbors face-to-face (Long 1986; Newbrough and Chavis 1986). A community fragmented by fear and mistrust, or exposed to undue hazards from inadequate housing, uncontrolled traffic, pollution, or violence, cannot be healthy, cannot establish the sense of cohesion needed to work for community development.

The affluent can buy services in protected enclaves, but only because others have already attended to the "good of all," creating an ecology and infrastructure to support public services and goods. Even the best protected enclaves are bought at the cost of freedom of movement, isolation from diversity, and overall decline in attachment and commitment to the wider society.

Attachment to place, to a geographic community, and attention to its needs beyond those of its separate residents—a sense of community responsibility based on a shared stake in a better future—is essential to sustain the environment that nurtures individuals and makes health and well-being possible. Regular and sustained contact, face-to-face and otherwise, are basic to trust, to the mutual recognition of common concerns and common ends, to the mutual identity that weaves the social fabric that ultimately sustains people (Susser 1993).

The Mission of Public Health

Traditionally, leaders in public health understood the importance of building and binding communities. They spoke out on the environmental essentials—the health-supporting infrastructure—for building health into the American future (Sigerist 1946). Preventing disease, prolonging life and promoting health requires not only health services but also the "development of social machinery which will ensure to every individual in the community a standard of living adequate for the maintenance of health" (Winslow 1926).

Public Responsibility for Health

Self-responsibility for health has its complement in a prior condition: the reservoir of community and public responsibility (Vickers 1984). Without collective responsibility—as expressed in a health-supporting environment that gives people options in housing, education, work, health, and child care—no one could "take responsibility for their own health."

Health services tools as embodied in current public policies, which center on the provision of health information and personal health services, are not likely to chart a course that leads away from the problems of disabled longevity and inequalities in health.

Health Information and Information for Health

People need information about what to do to be healthy—about lifestyle and other preventive and therapeutic behavior, timely access to appropriate health services, and the availability of both informal and organized support groups to provide emotional back-up, guidance, and material aid in critical life events. All this can be helpful when information is what individuals lack and when resources are available and accessible. Beyond this, and as important, is information to guide people to obtain everyday material resources—food, shelter, education, and income—and safe, secure environments that are essential for health.

But information itself is not enough for most people most of the the time to change their individual habits—no more than simple admonitions are enough to change the policymaking behavior of corporate decision makers, lawmakers, or health professionals (AHCPR 1992; Rochefort and Cobb 1993). Even newer psychosocial techniques for preventive health education, such as peer influence and skills training, are not enough in themselves to establish long-term changes in drug use, smoking and alcohol abuse, teen pregnancy, AIDS, or injuries (Elickson, Bell, and McGuigan 1993; Flay et al. 1989; Hansen 1992; Hayes 1987; Select Committee 1992; Robertson 1983; National Commission 1989; Kravitz et al. 1993; OTA 1991).

This failure of information and education has led to calls to change social and economic conditions, to develop resources that are needed to change risky living and change people's views of their tomorrows as uncertain, gray, and not worth attempting to plan for (Lanvin, Shapiro, and Weill 1992; Pentz et al. 1989; Perry et al. 1992; Haas et al. 1993; OTA 1991; Susser 1993).

This environmental and policy approach addresses organizations rather than individuals, because institutional impacts on health are more profound. Large organizations' decisions—most notably governments and corporations—affect the availability, quality, and distribution of essential health resources, ranging from health care, education, and jobs to food, housing, and environmental safety. They also affect the capacity of smaller organizations and individuals to participate in such decisions (OTA 1990; Milio 1986).

Information and Organization

Information serves more than the obvious but important purposes of creating awareness of issues, enhancing understanding and critical thinking, and recording and monitoring the past and present as a basis for action. When it is mutually exchanged, information also has communal uses. The two-way flow of information—whether face-to-face or through print and electronics—can also bind people, by fostering cohesion through common perspectives, common interests, and joint endeavors toward shared goals. This is eventually beneficial to the welfare of individual members of communities through material development of the community and its social fabric.

To the extent that information and communication serve to bind people and enable collective action, the development of new information technologies can become a facet in a health-supporting infrastructure that can help build healthy communities.

Health Care Reform

The necessary drive toward national health care reform of the 1990s will not of itself lead to sustainable health. The reform debate, by focusing on personal health services and their costs, sends an unspoken message to the public and politicians that health services equal health.

Effective universal access to health care can moderate some of the inequalities in health if disadvantaged groups and communities are given top priority. But the system of personal health services cannot deal very well with primary prevention, the avoidance of disabling and injurious illnesses. The important exceptions are few—birth control, immunizations, fluoride supplements, and to some extent, education about smoking cessation, sexual practices, diet, and injury prevention. Other clinical prevention tools are limited to secondary prevention—detecting existing problems and providing early intervention through screening and physical and laboratory examinations, such as prenatal care, mammography, blood pressure checks, and Pap smears (OTA 1993a; Milio 1983; Preventive Services Task Force 1989).

The less-favored social groups that have had least access to adequate care—those who pay most and get least in relative terms for the care they receive—being younger than the general population, can gain most from these public health services and should be first in line (AHCPR 1987). Even so, the impact will not be great enough to close the health gap with their advantaged counterparts, especially if they must copay for services. They are more likely than nonpoor people to delay or avoid care when they must pay a fee (OTA 1993b; Haas et al. 1993).

Clinical prevention, focusing on individuals, and the primary preventive potential of public health as embodied in its historic mission, focusing on organized community groups and populations, are complementary and would be most effective if they were restructured in a system to ensure collaboration in the future. But more is necessary and possible if there is to be progress toward healthy longevity and health equity.

Policy and Environment

The formal health care system tends to define health risks in rather narrow or technical ways (such as cigarette smoking or toxic pollutant levels), usually using specific probabilities that are independent of each other and separated from their context. Studies generally do not specify or give attention to the societal sources underlying risk indicators, focusing rather on those sources that are amenable to specific prevention and control techniques (Jasanoff 1990). It has been said that when all you have is a hammer, everything sooner or later begins to look invitingly like a nail (Gregory 1988).

Yet the litany of deficits in America's health-supporting social, economic, and physical environments clearly speaks to the importance of the complex societal web of public policies—fiscal, economic, education, technology, civil rights, labor, environmental, housing, social services, as well as health care—that shapes the prospects for the health of the nation, and especially of its more vulnerable groups. In today's world, policy is part of environment (Milio 1986).

Today the production of commercial and social goods and services in the United States is relying more on the transmission of information and less on energy than in any other century. Influence and power based on information, knowledge, and communication are becoming more important (Boyte 1991). This opens the possibility for people to become actors instead of reactors in public life, producers of programs and politics instead of consumers, partners and providers instead of clients and recipients of governments and large organizations.

Access to policymakers allows local groups to advocate for community health services, environmental safety, and improved housing, thus "empowering" groups to bring about community infrastructure development (Arterton 1984; Cook 1985; Smith 1988). But the increasingly prohibitive cost of entering the political arena, both locally and nationally, effectively excludes many small groups from being heard (Jasanoff 1990). Voices seeking to develop health-supporting infrastructures cannot compete with better financed, larger interests (Brown 1987; Minkler 1978; Murdoch and Goldberg 1989). Yet, with a supportive organizational base, they can be effectively heard (Lynn, Kartez, and Connelly 1992).

The costs of advocacy and community mobilization are much reduced by using the new information technologies in ways that link local, regional, and national groups, giving timely access to otherwise unavailable information. These technologies also enable public health agencies to develop mutually supportive ties with those groups, too long unheard, who want to build health into the future of their communities (Milio 1992).

A Renewed Public Health

The Institute of Medicine recently called on public health organizations to collaborate with the policy sectors of education, social services, housing, and income maintenance, explicitly recognizing that the origins of health and illness are tied to these policy sectors and are not within the control of individuals. People can only make responsible choices about their own health within the limits and opportunities set up in larger policy contexts (Institute of Medicine 1988).

If the public health community, in and outside of government, used a wider strategic vision than it has in recent years, it could take advantage of the new information technologies to create new "social machinery." Electronic linkages could connect them with diverse community groups, and they could engage in closer collaboration with organizational and policy sectors that shape people's health, the institutions that can address the primary prevention of chronic, disabling disease and injury, that enable the disabled, and that can end inequalities in health.

Information Technology and Health

Information, Referral, and Communication

Information technology can affect people's health in several ways. It can help individuals directly by giving them access to information about healthy living, about the prevention and treatment of illness, and about the availability of health services and health insurance. It can guide them to other sources of public and private assistance like training and education, food, fuel, and housing or job openings. Information technology can also connect them to on-line or other groups who have similar interests and problems. In other words, it provides information, referral, and communication.

Intelligence, Organization, and Advocacy

Information technology can affect people's health less directly and in broader, longer-lasting ways, given the limitations of information per se. These health effects occur through the use of information technology by the local and national organizations that sustain community life. Such groups include public health and health care organizations whose services can become more efficient and effective with information technology—for example, when they use electronic tools to streamline paperwork and make clinical and research knowledge available in timely, accurate, and confidential ways at all delivery sites; or when they upgrade training of personnel throughout the system and collaborate with other public and private organizations to develop programs and policies to promote health.

With information technology, other local organizations that supply health-supporting services—ranging from social services to housing, child care, youth, senior, and neighborhood resources—can similarly inform, guide, train, provide more effective services, mobilize, collaborate, and advocate for the community resources that are needed to support people's health.

In sum, information technology used by individuals and organizations can transmit information; conduct education, training, and research; improve service delivery; and enable communication, collaboration, mobilization, coalition building, and advocacy. All these activities can be done to create communities that are conducive to health. More effective than information and referral alone, intelligence (getting strategic information), organization, and advocacy—irrespective of distance, group size, or time limitations—also becomes possible.

The cases in the next section illustrate many of these ways to use information technology to support individuals and organizations for health-sustaining purposes, sometimes directly through health services and sometimes less directly through improving the conditions and quality of living.

New Health Care Systems

The prospect of more integrated health care systems offers a context for using IT in ways that go beyond typical, cost-saving administrative and clinical uses. Health organizations could also join more closely with community-based groups and engage in collaborative activities in new forms of relationships. In the changing delivery systems, guided by national standards and regulation and monitored by states, health programs will provide wider access to organized, least-cost health services through health maintenance organizations, home care, and other programs. The delivery systems will also be held accountable for the quality of services, including user satisfaction and cost control. Medically underserved communities especially will use community, school, and public health centers rather than hospitals; they will also need ancillary services, including transportation, outreach, translation, health education, social support, child care, and care for the homeless.

Health care systems will become electronically networked for administrative and professional clinical purposes. But the networks will focus on the wealthiest communities if compensatory policy does not address poor locales. These IT ties will also make possible, but not guarantee, new forms of cooperation for broader health-supporting purposes. Health departments and private health care systems, for example, if linked to each other, could also network with other community resources such as local Women, Infants, and Children's (WIC) food programs, and school health, occupational, and environmental programs. Beyond that, they could coordinate services with local or other public and private organizations responsible for health support, such as housing, employment, and training programs, child care arrangements, and income assistance services.

Information Technology and Health Services Delivery

The IT initiatives of community-based organizations in recent years suggest many other new and unimagined possibilities for collaboration with health services agencies, as the on-the-ground experiences of the people in Part II indicate. Families dealing with burdensome chronic health problems, for example, can be supported at home electronically by both health professionals and their own electronic support groups. At least 10 million people of all ages need constant attention to do their daily activities at home (GAO 1993b).

Mobile health teams, using wireless or notebook computers tied to health system servers and linked to community and regional networks, can provide direct care to the homeless wherever they congregate—in parks, at soup kitchens, and at shelters. Using a common database of available support services, the health teams could refer and facilitate access and transportation to sources of longer-term help. Similarly, visits could be made to migrant camps and church sites where people are reluctant or unable to go to formal health system facilities. Even small churches, with IT equipment, could offer emergency aid—to unemployed clients, for example, assessing their needs, referring them to health and other services, electronically checking eligibility for food stamps, unemployment insurance, and job training.

By establishing such cooperative electronic ties with community-based sites by barter or subcontract, health agencies could extend and strengthen their outreach in ways that are otherwise not possible. Health and other types of information and education could be transmitted from profession-operated sites, such as HMOs, universities, and voluntary agencies, to groups of students, teachers, staff, residents, and to people individually, in their homes and in school classrooms, child care centers, senior and youth centers, nursing homes, and libraries.

Using a variety of multimedia and two-way technology, a health agency could provide general information and education, staff training and updating, program planning, coordination of community health and safety campaigns, and early warning of environmental or occupational health problems—such as building hazards, infestations, toxic pollution, traffic or drug-related problems. Initiatives could also be taken from the community side among local participants to convey their concerns as a group to administrators and program monitors in health service systems.

These kinds of linkages would not only be cost-saving, but would also expand access to services and improve the quality of services by being more timely and responsive.

Public Health Agencies

National, state, and local public health agencies are planned to be wired among themselves before the end of the century, led by the federal Centers for Disease Control and Prevention (CDCP 1994). They should also begin wiring with relevant community agencies and organizations, ranging from local government, libraries, schools, and community health centers to community-sensitive churches, senior centers, and shelters. These connections would help them meet their mandate more effectively (see Figure 4.1).

The public health mandates are formally termed the "core functions" denoting "essential public health services" (see Figure 4.2) (Baker et al. 1993). The above examples suggest how electronic networks, through information, referral, and communication, can help fulfill public health functions of increasing access to personal health services, quality assurance, outreach, health education and information, training, and even improved monitoring and early warning of health-related problems in local environments and occupational sites. In addition, through electronic intelligence-gathering, organization, and advocacy, public health agencies could be more effective in their other less well-met tasks of community mobilization, leadership, and policy development. (Studnicki et al. 1994; Turnock et al. 1994; Zucconi and Carson 1994). These possibilities are not likely to be developed without national policy guidance and support.

Electronic networking, once begun, would spin off new variations, propelled by everyday community experience, moving from the obvious information and communication value of IT to new forms of organization, association, and action. As suggested in the case studies, the effect could be new, more participatory, flatter, and more effective relations between service providers in health care, education, social support, and governance. The new technology makes possible "community information technology." It moves from self-help, assistance, and mediated access to collaboration; it moves from information and referral to organized action.

Evaluating Health and Other Impacts of IT

No one has questioned either the need for or the appropriateness of public financing for research and development of information technology capacity in corporate, military, and government agencies, libraries,

Figure 4.1 Public Health and Community Electronic Networks

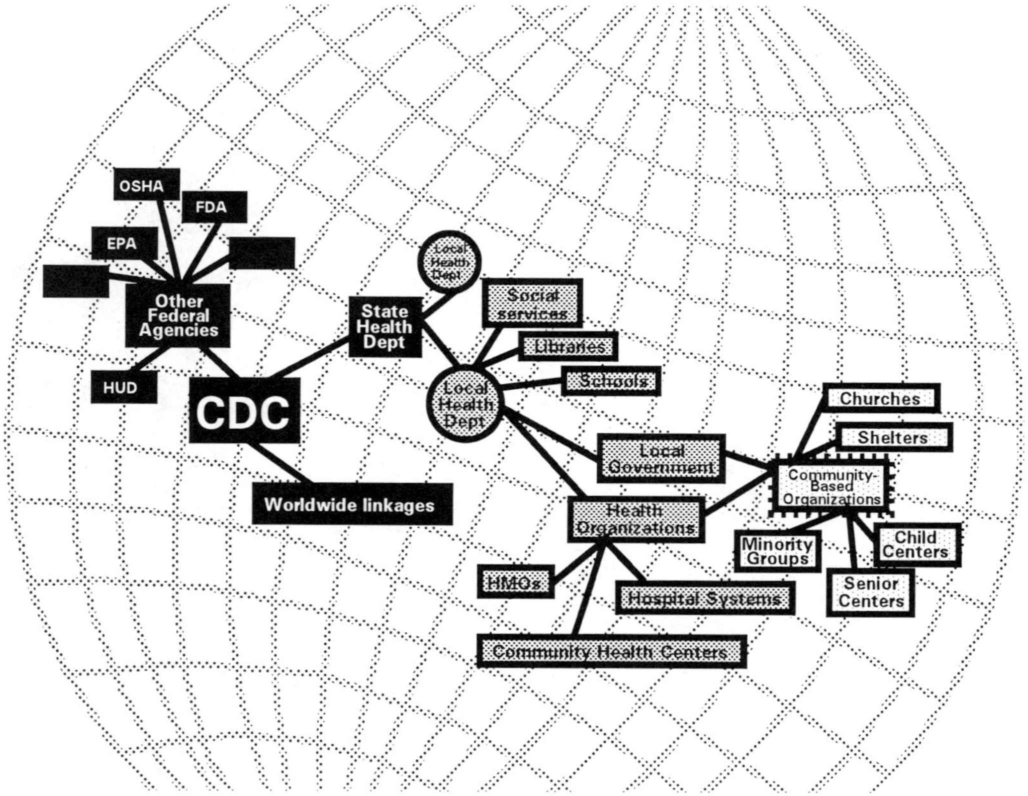

Figure 4.2 Essential Public Health Services

- Monitor health status to identify community problems.
- Diagnose and investigate community health problems and hazards.
- Inform, educate, empower people about health issues.
- Mobilize community partnerships and action to identify and solve health problems.
- Develop policies and plans that support individual and community health efforts.
- Enforce laws and regulations that protect health and ensure safety.
- Link people to needed personal health services and assure provision of health care when otherwise unavailable.
- Assure a competent public health and personal health care workforce.
- Evaluate effectiveness, accessibility, and quality of personal and population-based health services.
- Research for new insights and innovative solutions to health problems.

SOURCE: Essential Public Health Services Work Group of the Core Public Health Functions Steering Committee, American Public Health Association, September 1994.

schools, or health services. However, public policy support for extending information technology nets to community-based organizations and poor communities may well require "proof" of the need for and value of such action. At a minimum, evaluation of the effects of any such spending would be required. More importantly, many-sided evaluations, which are almost nonexistent to date, would serve as guides for further development of community information technology.

Almost all program evaluations focus on the information, education, and communications functions of information technology (evident in the reviews in Chapters 5, 7, 10, and 12). What do people seek and learn, from whom, and how often? Who are the users? The focus is almost exclusively on individual users. Generally, the answers show that people use communication more than information services; that there are far more readers than writers, far more receivers than senders; and that users are mainly more educated and affluent people, younger, and male. However, usage becomes shared more widely by others when public computer terminals are available.

Evaluations of information technology impacts on organizations are much less frequent. Studies have been done by and for corporations that are interested in cost-effectiveness (Thomas 1994). These studies usually focus on internal organizational structures and processes and do not address relations with other networked organizations (Schmitz and Fulk 1991; Kraemer et al. 1989).

Studies of the use of information technology by community-based organizations are rare. Findings suggest that small local organizations with information technology capacity serve as information intermediaries and advocates for their communities (Lynn and Koebrick 1994). But when deprived of information technology tools, they become increasingly less effective compared with their better-endowed counterparts (Murdock and Golding 1989). Virtually no studies have focused on information technology capacity development in low-budget community groups.

Evaluations of the connections between information technology and health also focus on individuals or on organizational cost-effectiveness, as reviewed in the next chapter. A broader picture of the impact of these technologies on health is needed, one that looks for the individual, organizational, and communitywide impacts on health and on the health-sustaining capacity of the community.

For individuals, this would mean learning about the personal and participatory uses of information technology, the changes in health status, and access to health and other needed services. For example, what information do individuals seek, both for health and other aspects of sustenance and quality of life; what sources do they use, and how do they use them; who are they and where do they access electronic information, education, referral, and communication services? As importantly, what are the less direct spin-offs of communication? Does collective activity develop in the form of "virtual organizations," face-to-face groups, and formal organizations? And for what purposes? Pleasure? Advocacy? Do the ends improve the health-supporting infrastructure of the community, whether in access to health services or in healthier living conditions?

Similar queries should be directed to IT-health connections among organizations, including conventional public health and health services agencies and health-supporting, small, community groups. Questions would address the sources and use of information and communication. But they would also focus on the secondary, spin-off effects involving the intelligence-gathering, organizing, and advocacy potential of information technology networks. The final questions would address successes and failures in bringing health-sustaining conditions into the communities. Here, interorganizational relations are important, as are changes within organizations and the development of new ones, new joint programs, and new coalitions.

Finally, at the community level, the questions would address whether the activities that were made possible and propelled by information technology among individuals and organizations are related to overall incidence and prevalence of disability, disease, death, and antecedent individual and community risk factors, such as smoking, unsafe sex, lack of housing, education, jobs, and health care. This scope of inquiry would require learning about the joint ventures among networked organizations, the effects on nonnetworked groups, and any changes in the practices, programs, and policies of agencies, businesses, and government resulting from the activities. As always, the failures, and the unwanted and unintended effects, should be sought out; these can be as helpful as learning from success.

No information technology impacts can be accepted as given. That is, a prior set of questions must be raised, especially in disadvantaged communities. How did the community groups develop their information technology capacity in the first place? With what resources and problems? What barriers and solutions? These are some of the questions asked in the cases presented in the next section.

Health-Secure Communities

The fundamental health problems in disadvantaged communities cannot be effectively addressed without improvements in health-supporting infrastructure beyond access to health services. One increasingly important component of that infrastructure is the IT capacity of community institutions. Community organizations can be a bridge in supporting one of the policy goals of the National Information Infrastructure: to prevent a new form of division between "haves" and "have-nots" (Brown 1993). The question is whether there is to be policy support to build up their IT capacity and close the gap between IT-poor and IT-rich organizations.

Public health in the twenty-first century could lead the way to health security, to a more disability-free longevity, and to health equity. If it can encompass in its strategic vision ways to promote new uses of the new electronic tools, especially among the diverse and often unheard voices in our communities—it may well find new allies and help create new "social machinery" to "assure the conditions in which people can be healthy."

References

Agency for Health Care Policy and Research (AHCPR). 1987. *National Health Expenditure Survey*. Washington, DC: DHHS.

———. 1992. *Information Dissemination to Health Care Practitioners and Policymakers.* Annotated Bibliography. Rockville, MD: USPHS, April.

American Dietetic Association. 1992. *Economic Benefits of Nutrition Services: Health Care Reform Legislative Platform.* Chicago, ADA.

Arterton, F. 1984. *Teledemocracy: Can Technology Protect Democracy?* Newbury Park, CA: Sage Publications.

Baker, E. L., R. J. Melton, P. V. Stange, M. L. Fields, J. P. Koplan, A. G. Fernando, and D. Satcher. 1993. "Health Reform and the Health of the Public: Forging Community Health Partnerships." *Journal of the American Medical Association* 272 (16): 1276–80.

Boyte, H. C. 1991. "Remapping Democratic Politics: Toward a Strong Version of Citizenship." History and Society Working Paper. University of Minnesota, Minneapolis, MN, 9 January.

Brenner, H., and A. Mooney. 1983. "Unemployment and Health in the Context of Economic Change." *Social Science & Medicine* 17 (16): 1125–38.

Brown, L. 1987. "Small Interventions for Large Problems: Reshaping Urban Leadership Networks." *Journal of Applied Science* 23 (2): 44–58.

Brown, R. 1993. *The National Information Infrastructure: Agenda for Action.* Washington, DC: U.S. Department of Commerce.

Calhoun, C. 1989. "Imagined Communities, Indirect Relationships and Postmodernism: Large Scale Social Integration and the Transformation of Everyday Life." Paper presented to the Conference on Social Theory and Emerging Issues in a Changing Society, Chicago, April 5–8.

Catalano R. 1991. "The Health Effects of Economic Insecurity." *American Journal of Public Health* 81 (9): 1148–52.

———. 1993. "Beyond Health Care: Economy and Public Health." Paper presented at the American Public Health Association Annual Meeting, San Francisco, 27 October.

Centers for Disease Control and Prevention (CDCP). 1994. "12 States Receive $4,335 Million and Join CDC's Information Network for Public Health Officials." Grant Summaries. Atlanta, GA: CDC, October.

Cook, R. 1995. "Predicting Arson." *BYTE* (February) 239–45.

Cowie, M., C. Fahrenbruch, L. Cobb, and A. Hallstrom. 1993. "Out-of-Hospital Cardiac Arrest: Racial Differences in Outcome in Seattle." *American Journal of Public Health* 83: 955–59.

Elickson, P., R. Bell, and K. McGuigan. 1993. "Preventing Adolescent Drug Use: Long-Term Results of a Junior High Program." *American Journal of Public Health* 83: 856–61.

Escarce, J., K. Epstein, D. Colby, and J. Schwarz. 1993. "Racial Differences in the Elderly's Use of Medical Procedures and Diagnostic Tests." *American Journal of Public Health* 83: 948–54.

Flay, B., D. Koepke, S. Thomson, et al. 1989. "Six Year Follow-up of the First Waterloo School Smoking Prevention Trial." *American Journal of Public Health* 79: 1371–6.

General Accounting Office. 1992a. *Early Intervention.* Washington, DC: U.S. Congress, 7 April.

———. 1992b. *Education Issues.* Washington, DC: U.S. Congress, December.

———. 1992c. *Environmental Protection Issues.* Washington, DC: U.S. Congress, December.

———. 1992d. *Housing Issues.* Washington, DC: U.S. Congress, December.

———. 1992e. *Investment Issues*. Washington, DC: U.S. Congress, December.

———. 1992f. *Labor Issues*. Washington, DC: U.S. Congress, December.

———. 1992g. *Poverty Trends, 1980–88: Changes in Family Composition and Income Sources among the Poor*. Testimony before the Subcommittee on Human Resources, Committee on Ways and Means, House of Representatives. Washington, DC: U.S. Congress, 10 September.

———. 1993a. *Decline in UI Beneficiaries*. Washington, DC: U.S. Congress, 7 October.

———. 1993b. Long-Term Care Forum. Discussion paper. Washington, DC: U.S. Congress, July.

———. 1993c. *Self-Sufficiency*. Washington, DC: U.S. Congress, August.

Gregory, B. 1988. *Inventing Reality*. New York: Wiley.

Gunning-Schepers, L. (ed.). 1990. *Socio Economic Inequalities in Health: Questions on Trends and Explanations*. The Hague: Dutch Ministry of Welfare, Health and Cultural Affairs.

Haas, J., S. Udvarhelyi, C. Morris, and A. Epstein. 1993. "The Effect of Providing Health Coverage to Poor Uninsured Pregnant Women in Massachusetts." *Journal of the American Medical Association* 269 (1): 87–91.

Hansen, W. 1992. "School-Based Substance Abuse Prevention: A Review of the State of the Art in Curriculum, 1980–1990." *Health Education Research* 7: 403–30.

Hayes, C. D., (ed.). 1987. *Risking the Future: Adolescent Sexuality, Pregnancy, and Childbearing*. Washington, DC: National Academy Press.

Hogue, C., and M. Hargraves. 1993. "Class, Race, and Infant Mortality in the United States." *American Journal of Public Health* 83: 9–12.

Howard, J., B. Hankey, R. Greenberg, et al. 1992. "A Collaborative Study of Differences in the Survival Rates of Black Patients and White Patients with Cancer." *Cancer* 69: 2349–60.

Hutchins, S., J. Gindler, W. Atkinson, et al. 1993. "Preschool Children at High Risk for Measles: Opportunities to Vaccinate." *American Journal of Public Health* 83: 862–67.

Institute of Medicine. 1988. *The Future of Public Health*. Washington, DC: National Academy Press.

———. 1991. *The Computer-based Patient Record: An Essential Technology for Health Care*. Washington, DC: National Academy Press.

Jasanoff, S. 1990. *The Fifth Branch Science Advisers as Policymakers*. Cambridge, MA: Harvard University Press.

Joint Economic Committee. 1984. *Economic Change, Physical Illness, and Social Deviance*. Committee Print 98-200. Washington, DC, U.S. Congress, 72–110.

Jones, H. 1956. "A Special Consideration of the Aging Process, Disease and Life Expectancy." *Advances In Biological and Medical Physics* 4: 281–337.

Kaplan, G. A., and R. Camacho. 1983. "Perceived Health and Mortality: A Nine-Year Follow-Up of the Human Population Laboratory Cohort." *American Journal of Epidemiology* 117: 292–308.

Keeney, R. 1980. "Mortality Rates Induced by Economic Expenditures." *Risk Analysis* 10 (1): 150–54.

Kennedy, P. 1993. *Preparing for the 21st Century*. New York: Random House.

Kottke, T. 1986. "Disease and Risk Factor Clustering in the U.S.: Implications for Public

Health Policy." In Office of Disease Prevention and Health Promotion, *Integration of Risk Factor Interventions*, 1–62. Washington, DC: U.S. Department of Health and Human Services.

Kraemer, K. L., L. King, N. E. Dunkle, and J. P. Lane. 1989. *Managing Information Systems: Change and Control in Organizational Computing*. San Francisco: Jossey-Bass.

Kravitz, R., et al. 1993. "Recall of Recommendations and Adherence to Advice among Patients with Chronic Medical Conditions." *Archives of Internal Medicine* 153: 1869–78.

Landrigan, P. 1992. "Environmental Disease—Preventable Epidemic." *American Journal of Public Health* 82: 941–43.

Lanvin, A., G. Shapiro, and K. Weill. 1992. "Creating an Agenda for School-Based Health Promotion: A Review of Selected Reports." Cambridge, MA: Harvard School of Public Health.

Lieu, T., P. Newacheck, and M. McManus. 1993. "Race, Ethnicity, and Access to Ambulatory Care among U.S. Adolescents." *American Journal of Public Health* 83: 960–65.

Long, N. 1986. "The City as a Political Community." *Journal of Community Psychology* 14: 72–80.

Louv, R. 1985. *America II*. New York: Penguin.

Lynn, F., and A. Koebrick. 1994. Communities, Sustainable Development and the National Information Infrastructure. Chapel Hill, NC: University of North Carolina, August.

Lynn, F., J. Kartez, and C. Connelly. 1992. *The Toxics Release Inventory: Environmental Democracy in Action*. Washington, DC: Environmental Protection Agency, January.

Marmot, M., and M. McDonnell. 1986. "Mortality Decline and Widening Social Inequalities." *Lancet* (2): 274–76.

McKinlay, J., S. McKinlay, R. Beaglehole. 1989. "A Review of the Evidence Concerning the Impact of Medical Measures on Recent Mortality and Morbidity in the United States." *International Journal of Health Services* 19 (2): 181–208.

Merva, M., and R. Fowles. 1992. *Effects of Diminished Economic Opportunities on Social Stress: Heart Attacks, Strokes, and Crime*. Paper published by the Economic Policy Institute, University of Utah, Salt Lake City, October.

Meyerowitz, J. 1985. *No Sense of Place: The Impact of Electronic Media on Social Behavior*. New York: Oxford.

Milio, N. 1983. *Primary Care and the Public's Health: Judging Impacts, Goals and Policies*. Lexington, MA: Lexington/Heath.

———. 1986. *Promoting Health Through Public Policy*. Ottawa: Canadian Public Health Association.

———. 1991. "Toward Healthy Longevity: Lessons in Food and Nutrition Policy Development from Finland and Norway." *Scandinavian Journal of Social Medicine* 19 (2): 209–17.

———. 1992. "New Tools for Community Development in Health." *Health Promotion International* 7 (3): 207–19.

Minkler, M. 1978. "Ethical Issues in Community Organization." *Health Education Monograph* 6 (2): 198–209.

Montgomery, L. 1992. *Increased Effects of Poverty on the Health of U.S. Children and*

Young People Since 1976. Paper presented at the Annual Meeting of the American Public Health Association, Washington, DC, 9 November.

Muller, A. 1992. *The Business Cycle and Community Hospitals Admissions*. Paper presented at the American Public Health Association, Washington, DC, November.

Murdock, G., and P. Golding. 1989. "Information, Poverty and Political Inequality: Citizenship in the Age of Privatized Communications." *Journal of Communication* 39 (3): 180–85.

National Commission for Injury Prevention and Control. 1989. *Injury Prevention: Meeting the Challenge*. New York: Oxford University Press.

Newbrough, J., and D. Chavis. 1986. "Psychological Sense of Community." *Journal of Community Psychology* 14: 3–5.

Office of Technology Assessment. 1986. *Technology and Structural Unemployment: Reemploying Displaced Adults*. Washington, DC: U.S. Congress.

———. 1990. *Critical Connections*. Washington, DC: U.S. Congress, January.

———. 1991. *Adolescent Health* 1 (26).

———. 1992. *Does Health Insurance Make a Difference*? Washington, DC: U.S. Congress, 15 September.

———. 1993a. *Benefit Design: Clinical preventive services*. Washington, DC: U.S. Congress, September.

———. 1993b. *Benefit Design: Patient Cost-Sharing*. Washington, DC: U.S. Congress, September.

———. 1993c. *International Health Statistics: What Do They Mean for the United States*? Washington, DC: U.S. Congress, November.

Olshansky, S., M. Rudberg, B. Carnes, C. Cassel, and J. Brody. 1991. "Trading Off Longer Life for Worsening Health: The Expansion of Morbidity Hypothesis." *Journal of Aging and Health* 3 (2): 194–216.

Oswald, J. 1988. "Overview of New Medical Technology." *Strategic Planning Analysis*. Minneapolis, MN: Group Health.

Pentz, M., J. Dwyer, D. Mackinnon, et al. 1989. "A Multi-Community Trial for Primary Prevention of Adolescent Drug Abuse: Effects on Drug Use Prevalence." *Journal of the American Medical Association* 261: 3259–66.

Perry, C., S. Kelder, D. Murray, and K. Klepp. 1992. "Community-wide Smoking Prevention: Long-term Outcomes of the Minnesota Heart Health Program and the Class of 1989 Study." *American Journal of Public Health* 82: 1210–16.

Preventive Services Task Force. 1989. *Guide to Clinical Preventive Services: An Assessment of the Effectiveness of 169 Interventions*. Baltimore, MD: Williams and Wilkins.

Rice, D., and M. LaPlante. 1986. *The Burden of Multiple Chronic Conditions: Past Trends and Policy Implications*. Presented at the Annual Meeting of the American Public Health Association, Las Vegas.

Robertson, L. 1983. *Injury Control*. Lexington, MA: Lexington Press.

Rochefort, D., and R. Cobb. 1993. "Problem Definition, Agenda Access, and Policy Choice." *Policy Studies Journal* 21 (1): 56–71.

Rogers, R. 1992. "Living and Dying in the U.S.A.: Sociodemographic Determinants of Death Among Blacks and Whites." *Demography* 29 (2): 287–303.

Roos, N., and B. Havens. 1991. "Predictors of Successful Aging: A Twelve-Year Study of Manitoba Elderly." *American Journal of Public Health* 81: 63–68.

Rosenfeld, A. 1978. *New Views of Older Lives*. Washington, DC: National Institute of Mental Health.

Sale, K. 1993. "The U.S. Green Movement Today." *Nation* (July): 92–96.

Schmitz, J., and J. Fulk. 1991. "Organizational Colleagues, Media Richness, and Electronic Mail: A Test of the Social Influence Model of Technology Use." *Communication Research* 18 (4): 487–523.

Select Committee on Children, Youth, and Families. 1992. *A Decade of Denial in Teens and AIDS in America*. Washington, DC: U.S. Congress.

Sigerist, H. E. 1946. *The University at the Crossroads: Addresses and Essays*. New York: Henry Schuman.

Smith, L. 1988. "The Development of Computer Applications by Non-Employed People in Community Settings." *Journal of Occupational Psychology* 61 (1): 89–102.

Smith, R. 1987. *Unemployment and Health*. New York: Oxford University Press.

Steckel, R. 1989. "Heights and Health in the United States, 1710–1912." In *Auxology 88: Perspectives in the Science of Growth and Development*, edited by J. Tanner. London: Smith-Gordon, Ltd.

Studnicki, J., B. Steverson, H. N. Blais, E. Goley, T. B. Richards, and J. N. Thornton. 1994. "Analyzing Organizational Practices in Local Health Departments" *Public Health Reports* 109 (4): 485–88.

Susser, M. 1993. "Health as a Human Right: An Epidemiologist's Perspective on Public Health." *American Journal of Public Health* 83: 481–84.

Suzman, R. 1988. *Population Epidemiological Research Highlights FY 1988*. Washington, DC: National Institute on Aging, 25 April.

Thomas, R. 1994. *What Machines Can't Do*. Berkeley: University of California Press.

Turnock, B. J., A. Handler, W. Hall, S. Potsic, R. Nalluri, and E. H. Vaughn. 1994. "Local Health Department Effectiveness in Addresing the Core Functions of Public Health." *Public Health Reports* 109 (5): 653–58.

Verbrugge, L. M. 1985. "Gender and Health: An Update on Hypotheses and Evidence." *Journal of Health and Social Behavior* 26: 156–82.

Vickers, G. 1984. *Human Systems Are Different*. New York: Harper & Row.

Wescott, A., H. Vollmer, and G. Svensson. 1985. *Health Policy Implications of Unemployment*. Copenhagen: WHO, Regional Office for Europe.

Williams, D. 1990. "Socioeconomic Differentials in Health: A Review and Redirection." *Social Psychology Quarterly* 53 (2): 81–99.

Winslow, C. 1926. *The Evolution and Signficance of the Modern Public Health Campaign*. New Haven: Yale University Press.

Zucconi, S. L., and C. A. Carson. 1994. CDC's Consensus Set of Health Status Indicators: Monitoring and Prioritization by State Health Departments. *American Journal of Public Health* 84 (10): 1644–48.

PART

II

Case Studies in Community Information Technology

INTRODUCTION TO PART II

EACH OF the five cases in this section is preceded by a chapter giving an overview of published and unpublished studies, to provide background and perspective to the general area of concern: health care, welfare, education, economic development, and participatory governance.

Health Care

The selective review of health care reports on information technology in Chapter 5 suggests that a leap in thinking is needed among many medical professionals to see and appreciate the organizing and community services potential of information technology.

Chapter 6 addresses support for home caregivers of chronically ill family members through electronic networks tied to both professionals, community organizations, and other caregivers. These uses of information technology reveal the potential health benefits of electronic information, referral, and communication with supportive peers and professionals.

The case also illustrates some information technology program development processes: grant-getting strategies, how professionals respond when they think their turf is being threatened, and the process of adapting medical information to make it user-friendly for ordinary people. It demonstrates the problems of maneuvering the vague line between collaboration and competition that often exists in academic and other professional organizations, especially in an era of scarce resources.

The chapter shows too, through the contrasts of the networked AIDS and Alzheimer's programs, that the viability of community information technology requires an organized nexus in which it can be embedded. Finally, the unintended spin-offs from CareNet suggest not only new kinds of individual responses to IT, but also new kinds of organization.

Community Welfare

Chapter 7 is a review of literature on the uses of information technology by school children and elders. It shows that it will take more than placing equal numbers of computers in schools to assure IT equity among school districts, schools, ethnic and language groups, and genders. The IT capacity of poorer schools needs special support, including better software, more qualified teachers and computer-related texts, funds for machine repair, technical support, and retraining. The review also shows that newly computer-literate elders are helping other adults and children learn to use computers. They donate computer time and services to community groups or individuals, write club reports, and provide computer support for nonprofit organizations like food aid groups, libraries, and churches.

The two cases that follow (Chapters 8 and 9) reveal laborious but successful efforts in two communities to link age groups in a neighborhood and reach out to support those who are cast out of the mainstream of community life.

The first case takes place in problem-ridden Southcity, where an ecumenical group of churches coordinate a comprehensive range of social and health services through a local electronic network and database for the purposes of information, referral, and intergroup communication. Among the members is a hospital system that delivers ambulatory care through mobile teams equipped with laptop computers. This story suggests how health care and health-supporting services can be coordinated and delivered with information technology and the price that will be paid by some disadvantaged people when local or national organizational politics exclude them. At the same time, it suggests that when required by the carrot of federal funding, contentious groups are often able to find grounds for compromise.

The potential leadership of elders in community information technology shows up in Chapter 9, the story of Midcity. There, retirees set up a computer learning center and other programs in disadvantaged areas. Important ingredients in the effort were local and federal government support, IT developments in city and school services, friendly ties with the local university, the public-private sponsored "freenet," the marketing interests of local ophthalmologists, and the solid social ties of the elders who were connected to all these activities. The case reveals how both necessity and opportunity can become the mother of invention. It also shows that organizational collaboration is based on organizations' views of their interests, and is stronger when they share mutual interests. The result in Midcity was especially fruitful cooperation.

Economic and Community Development

Some of the local job development and distance learning aspects of community information technology are set out in Chapter 10. Early reports suggest that IT centers for work or learning (or both) have many of the advantages of home-based methods and fewer of the disadvantages, such as isolation and distractions. Whether begun by governments, corporations, or public-private partners, or by departments of transportation, commerce, rural development, or education, the results are similar. Planning and support and phased-in voluntary participation for appropriate job types are important elements, and cost savings and employee and client satisfaction are among the benefits.

In Europe, where half the population still lives outside major metropolitan areas, "teleservice centers" or "electronic village halls" began more than a decade ago. There are many variants (over 120 in Finland and Norway alone) in forms "somewhere between a coffeehouse and a post office." A consensus is emerging that in order to operate within budget or at a profit the centers have to be responsive to local needs and to be networked in a cooperative relationship with other centers.

Development of a telebusiness center in rural England's Hill Park is the focus of Chapter 11. It offers several contrasts with other more socially oriented centers that address broader information and education concerns. The mix of English "telecottages" is reflected in their telecottage association, an important vehicle for the development and support of member centers. Responding to the constraints and opportunities they faced, the telecottages came to be a balance between community development—nurturing local groups, schools, churches, and the disadvantaged—and economic development—supporting local businesses and bringing in work and jobs. All of these local institutions underpin the quality of life and health in the community.

Democratic Electronic Decision Making

The review of information technology in a participatory democracy (Chapter 12) notes that in the past, the opportunity for input often came in the form of limited, one-way, passive participation. With the emerging new technologies the future of public participation in government is still uncertain. Reports show that the depth of public interest, the opportunity and incentives to participate in policy processes at any level of public life, varies widely but favors certain economic and educational groups. To correct this imbalance all citizens need access to the hardware, software, the skills and navigational tools to find and use the benefits of the electronic world, to access the new tools in ways comparable to the old penny press, universal phone service, and the free broadcast media of previous decades.

The final case (Chapter 13) illustrates how electronic democracy worked with homeless people in the affluent city of Westsun. The city had all the essential ingredients for initiating community IT: elected leaders with a history of participatory governance, competent staff, and interested, idea-prone citizens. Unanticipated results suggest the potential of broad-based information technology for bringing about health-supporting conditions in communities.

Lessons

Chapter 14 explores the cross-cutting themes and issues from the cases and draws some lessons in preparation for Part III, where policy implications are developed.

SECTION A

New Ways to Deliver Health Services

[Public health is] *The science and art of preventing disease, prolonging life, and promoting physical and mental health and efficiency through organized community efforts, for the sanitation of the environment, the control of community infections, the education of the individual in the principles of personal hygiene, the organization of medical and nursing service for the early diagnosis and treatment of disease, and the* **development of social machinery which will ensure to every individual in the community a standard of living adequate for the maintenance of health.**

C.E.A. Winslow, *The Evolution and Significance of the Modern Public Health Campaign*, 1926

CHAPTER

5

HEALTH SERVICES DELIVERY USING INFORMATION TECHNOLOGY

From Provider Control toward Consumer Support

THE GLITTERING world of information technologies portrayed by the commercial press has often proved chimerical when pursued by real people. By contrast, thinking about information technology (IT) in the health field has been too narrow. Well into the nineties, there was little effort to explore the possibilities of IT beyond delivering text and numerical data, sound, and images. The qualitative leap to looking at the organizing potential of IT was largely outside the line of vision of principal policymaking groups. Organization requires not only communication, but also coordination, collaboration, leadership, and effective decision making, all of which can be done on electronic pathways. A brief survey of the issues that have concerned health care providers and policymakers in the nineties, ranging from uses of IT in and outside of hospitals and as supports to practitioners and patients, give a backdrop to the broader and more imaginative activities depicted in the first case.

The uses of IT in health care, evident in the literature and reports reviewed here, have largely centered on extending conventional information and communication to support mainly administrative rather than service delivery tasks and providers rather than consumers or community-based organizations. This focus is likely to remain, but the scope will widen, if slowly, because social, political, and economic pressures will require it.

Policy Issues

Technology

The administrative and provider focus of policymakers and analysts lead them to address the technical and fiscal hurdles to a smoothly working electronic web. These problems have included the development of information and electronic standards to which all parties adhere, and technical improvements, such as very friendly user interfaces accessible by pen or voice, new data management and security systems, and higher speeds for wireless (cellular and satellite) data networks. Many of these issues will be resolved under national leadership to bring about consensus among large-scale stakeholders in government, business, and the health professions.

Beyond the technological and financial issues attached to IT development are other policy matters related to the information itself and how to manage it. How much should be available; who should have access to it; how will people give informed consent and be able to correct, add, or delete personal information (related to mental, sexual, or genetic conditions) that could affect future employer decisions (OTA 1993). Errors in medical records are well-known (Chan and Schonfield 1992). Without safeguards, the numbers of observers would grow exponentially. These ethical issues will have to be weighed against other interests, such as cost accounting, legal documentation, regulatory monitoring, and research (Detmer and Steen 1993). Virtually all of the public will be affected, yet few are even aware of the issues, much less have a basis for understanding the implications or an effective channel to develop and raise their views.

One solution to privacy issues is found in many western European countries, which have universal health care programs. It is the "smart card," which is similar to a credit card encoded with a variety of information ("Overview" 1993; Pangalos 1992). This could include health insurance data, medical history, emergency health information such as blood type, and medical prescriptions. The information on the card can be separated in ways that allow access only by specific information to specific health workers. A pharmacist, for example, could access only prescription data, but would also need a "key" to unlock it. Alternatively, the smart card might only allow access to a central data file, one kept by a person's health care system and openable only by a dual "key" card held by the appropriate practitioner or authorized person. A range of smart card pilot tests were started in almost half the states in the United States by the mid-nineties (OTA 1993).

Creating interoperable hardware and software for health services is a vast undertaking, a component of the information technology industry valued at about $5 billion annually. But more than commercial interests are at stake (OTA 1993). Policies on technical issues, once resolved, will affect the shape of health care delivery in major ways. The arrangements will determine the accessibility of health services and health information to patients and the general public. Yet there is no easy way for the millions who will be affected by the policy decisions to raise their voices in stakeholder forums because they are dispersed and unorganized.

The number, fluidity, and complexity of the issues mean that policy decisions about health care IT will be continually informed and revised as all parties gain on-the-ground experience.

The Imperatives of Health Care Delivery

Efficient and effective systems of care require standardized forms and data sets, documentation of clinical services, the development of privacy controls, and ready access to selected information at all sites where services are provided. Network computers and other developing electronic technologies provide essential support for these tasks. As health services organizations become more intertwined and mutually dependent, new attempts are being made to use IT to improve health care efficiency and effectiveness, which must include reaching underserved groups, satisfying patients, and improving patients' health. All of this implies cost. New public- and private-sector mandates for access and quality provide an incentive to use new methods, including IT, to meet these demands in cost-effective ways.

The pressure to control costs also limits the time providers spend with patients. Doctors and nurses spend from a third to half of their time writing up patient charts (Institute of Medicine 1991). The case for using IT to automate patient records was graphically posed by a General Accounting Office estimate showing that the yearly 34 million hospital admissions and 1.2 billion visits to physicians generated 10 billion pages of medical records (GAO 1993).

There is also growing interest in using IT as a new patient or consumer resource for clinical information because health professionals often do not always communicate well with their clients in face-to-face encounters (International Medical Benefits 1993). Professionals will not necessarily be available when and where they are needed because cost-containment pressures will continue to restrict their time.

Making the Conventional Better: Provider Support

These imperatives have given momentum to the search for better ways to use IT in health services delivery, if mainly along familiar paths. Well into the nineties, using information technology to deliver health services meant providing support to health care practitioners, physicians, nurses and others at the bedside, sometimes in nursing homes and clinics, but only occasionally in the community (Gogdetz 1985). Supporting public health through IT was relatively rare or limited in scope.

Information

It is no surprise that the first and still primary use of the proliferating electronic infrastructure in health care is the development, processing, storage, and transmission of information. It is one solution to contemporary "information overload" in medicine and health. In the last ten years, the numbers of journals and health organizations that disseminate health services information has more than doubled. There are over 1,300 federal and state health agencies and 1,800 research centers that produce health information as part of their mission. An additional 850 commercial firms publish and provide computerized health information (Harris Consulting 1994).

Hospitals

Although IT has the potential to support new ways to deliver health services and improve health, administrative support has remained the main task for electronic information technologies and the prime hope for cost savings in the move toward managed care reforms and wider access to care.

One community hospital in California, for example, pioneered a comprehensive medical information system in the early 1970s, computerizing clinical information from patient admission to completion of treatment. Within three years it was saving \$3 to \$5 per patient day, or about a half-million dollars a year, almost all from saving nursing time otherwise spent with chart-related paperwork. Savings quadrupled in the eighties, as IT costs declined and labor costs increased (AHCPR 1992a). Another hospital system claimed to save \$900 per patient when it required physicians to use computerized patient records before ordering drugs or tests, avoiding costly drug reactions and duplicate testing ("Technology Payoff" 1993). Hospital-based nurses were able to effectively decide over the telephone the best avenue of care for AIDS patients—whose treatment cost more than \$100,000 throughout their illness—when assisted by a computerized program that guided the interview (AHCPR 1992b; U.S. Congress 1992; Evans et al. 1993).

The most frequent and avid adopters of sophisticated IT systems were large hospitals and health care systems, tying together HMOs and other service units with health insurers. They emphasized data analysis capabilities to gain efficiencies and improve profit margins in the for-profit systems. This meant profiling utilization patterns of physicians to get physician "bill-busters," to identify attractive patient markets (the "pool and patio" clients), and to estimate the odds of survival of critical care patients in order to move them to less-expensive beds—or to avoid more costly treatment in intensive care units when the odds of survival were slim (Reichard 1993).

Practitioner Support

Information technology support for practitioners comes in the form of electronic information, education, and communication to help assess and diagnose, treat, and monitor the progress of the patients who go to physician offices.

Computerized databases can remind physicians to contact their patients to make a visit for routine prevention services such as influenza vaccinations. In some situations these reminders have reduced hospital care by up to 30 percent in one winter season (McDonald and Tierney 1992). Electronic alerts also reminded them about potential drug reactions when they prescribed medications, and helped them determine the appropriate antibiotic rather than delaying treatment until laboratory culture tests were completed (Evans et al. 1993).

One commercial computer network automated medical and insurance claims data for office-based physicians, charging about $3,000 a year in the early nineties for leased hardware, software, and user support services. It included linkages with other health care delivery sites, insurers, and medical information services. To enhance its profit margin, the firm required doctors to view several dozen drug advertisements, take four continuing education programs per year, and allow the vendor to access the physicians' patient data in the aggregate and use it as a marketing research database to sell to researchers and medical product manufacturers (Physician Computer Network 1992).

Provider Education

To extend support to doctors and nurses in rural areas as well as patients who had access to a networked computer, a university medical center in Texas initiated a computer network to offer low-cost multimedia continuing education. The self-paced computer programs included mental health, maternal and child health, and treating and caring for trauma patients (Ramirez 1991; Petryshen and Pelekis 1992).

In rural India, where health professionals are sparse, computers have supported local, village-based community health workers by guiding their development of work plans, providing updated information for the health advice they gave to patients, serving as a database for patient records, and monitoring their services from a centrally located health care facility (Nath and Tuli 1991).

The Public Health Council in North Carolina tested a new way to educate its new board of health members located in dispersed rural counties. Through a satellite teleconference network based in local facilities, it held a series of sessions in which participants could also call in to a central panel of experts and join in the subject under discussion (Association of Boards 1991).

Problems

Although there is great potential for IT to improve practitioner services, the reality may be otherwise without a supportive environment. In London, for example, in a program linking solo practitioners to hospital computers, doctors avoided using their computers basically because the network was not easily interoperable. The record systems, among other things, were incompatible (Aird 1992).

In Australia, where a third of doctors used computers for fiscal management, only 2 to 14 percent used IT for clinical purposes such as reminders for preventive care, getting drug information, or reviewing the medical literature. A survey concluded that government funds should support broader and more effective uses by clinicians, a majority of whom voiced interest in finding new ways to use the technology (Commonwealth 1992).

Relatively few nurses have used bedside computers to care for medical and obstetric patients. Like other health professionals in the nineties, many have had little experience with computers and so have also not been comfortable using them for day-to-day paperwork. Extensive training will be needed to enable the potential uses of IT in health care delivery to become reality within the foreseeable future. As a profession, nursing has focused on developing informatics, the database elements appropriate to providing nursing services (National Center for Nursing Research 1993; Brennan and Fitzpatrick 1993).

Outside Hospital Walls

Attempts to use information technology in health services outside of hospitals were minimal until well into the nineties.

Home Care and Community Health Providers

To support its community health nurses, one agency proposed an IT system to help nurses address the problems of their elderly homebound patients. Using an electronic network, the nurse would communicate with a clinical nurse specialist and other on-line consultants who might suggest an article to read. The nurse could then search the database for the article, and read or print out the abstract, among other possibilities (Hekelman, Niles, and Brennan 1993). Other computer programs have been designed to help community nurses do "community nursing diagnosis" (Wright 1985).

To save time and ensure accurate records, British home visit nurses tested computerized files long before handheld devices were developed (Harrison and Green 1986). But American entrepreneurs in the home care industry rapidly adopted portable IT during the same period, motivated by profit prospects. Each day, staff nurses would download the agency's patient records through a telephone link to portable computers. The staff then entered data in the homes during service visits, and at the end of the day they transmitted the records by phone to the host computer. There, new treatments or other information could be automatically updated and necessary reports on services, quality, and billing were generated (Klein 1993).

As a result of this technology, as well as hiring more home health aides and providing more technology-intensive services such as infusion therapy, profit-making home care companies were able to increase their market share by two-thirds in less than a decade (Klein 1993). A further incentive to use information technology in all home health agencies occurred in the early nineties. A congressional rule shortened the reimbursement time for delivered Medicare services if agencies used electronic claims processing; the software was provided free of charge. Paper-based claims took twice as long and could not be electronically deposited in an agency's bank (Klein 1993).

In one state health department in the mid-1980s, public health nurses created a workable computerized community-focused system for planning and monitoring services. But, after several efforts, the leadership and support needed to implement it could not be found (Kosidlak and Kerpelman 1987).

Public health agencies, the state and local health departments that have statutory mandates to oversee the health of the people in their jurisdictions, typically have used information technology for administrative and planning purposes, and have developed databases for monitoring services and the health status of their populations (Hodge and Steele 1991; Bliss, Foster, and Ho 1991; Scheske 1991). The federal Centers for Disease Control and Prevention began new efforts in the nineties to make large health databases freely available in increasingly user-friendly formats to local public health professionals and others, and began to consider uses of IT beyond wider access to information (Friede, Reid, and Ory 1993).

Community-Based Pharmacy

Another spur to moving medical information into the community was a 1993 federal law covering prescribed drugs, which encouraged new uses of IT in pharmacies across the country. All pharmacists must offer to discuss drug information with patients and family members, especially how and when to use the drugs and any side effects (Omnibus 1990). Computerized programs now contain not only technical drug data but also formats that are consumer-friendly, including printouts with personalized directions. To entice pharmacists to buy the IT systems, some of these include advertisements from drug manufacturers in the form of printout coupons for over-the-counter brand name drugs. Other variations include computer kiosks located in the pharmacy's public space, which consumers can use at will, and which display ads over the screens. Some of these programs also contain information on illnesses, lifestyle, and self-health appraisals (Barker, Allan, and Swensson 1989).

Community-Provider Connections

In a demonstration designed to move beyond IT support for large-scale health care providers, an electronic net in the Capitol includes child development centers and homeless shelters among its initial 15 sites. The project aims to coordinate health and human services locally and to learn whether this would improve the health-effectiveness of the activities. The network offers a services directory of over 600 agencies and the capacity to hold multiparty video conferences and enable a practitioner to talk with a patient at a distant location.

This community approach to delivering services has an individual focus—case management. The client data can, for example, be "eco-mapped"—showing the person's support system of contacts with a variety of agencies, and his or her family tree. What is missing is the larger picture, an "ecology" of the organized resources in the community that could contribute to community-wide prevention of the kinds of problems—such as drugs or unwanted pregnancies or heart disease—that brought the individual to the practitioner (Public Health Service 1993).

In more problematic circumstances in the coalfields of West Virginia, a six-agency coalition obtained computer hardware and financing but were unable to implement their IT network plans. They wanted to provide computer network–assisted training and support for outreach workers to deliver community development, health, and welfare services to rural communities. One reason for seeking computer communications was the fact that rural telephone service was not reliable. But the lack of telephone service itself prevented formation of the interagency computer network, along with a lack of time and expertise to create workable software (Couto 1986). Obviously, IT without technical support and basic community resources cannot build communities.

Beyond Providers: Consumer Support

Self-Help for Individuals

In the mid-1980s, Cleveland's free electronic network included a kind of "electronic hospital and information dispensary" for computer users. The information and communications program was made as user-friendly as possible. The core of the system was its "medical clinic." By selecting this option, a user could read or anonymously post a question related to medical care. Family physicians monitored the system and answered questions. They did no diagnosing or treating, but they gave general information on any topics that arose, much as they would in their own offices (Grunder and Garrett 1986).

Computer-based self-health appraisal forms seem to connote a nonjudgmental vehicle that encourages young people to "talk" about sensitive topics like sex and sexual abuse. Studies of teens and young adults show that when they provide information to a computer, they become willing to follow printout advice or discuss issues more openly with a medical advisor. As a result, some young people have changed their attitudes toward AIDS prevention and birth control, although whether their behavior has changed is not known. College students too have followed their computers' advice and managed their own simpler health problems, reducing visits to the campus clinic (Paperny et al. 1990; Paperny and Starn 1989; Thomas, Cahill, and Durlak 1993; Anderson 1988; Robinson and Walters 1987).

Similar computer-based educational programs for patients with chronic diseases and people who want to quit smoking are able to help individuals learn about their health problem and guide them in making necessary changes. The results are about as good as most other methods, such as counseling, reading, or group work, but have the advantages of being under the immediate time-control of the user and being cost-effective for the health care delivery system (Ellis 1987; Schneider 1986).

Newer software programs that have become available to consumers in the 1990s offer a richer menu of ways to individualize information than was previously available. One computer-based system for people living with AIDS/HIV, for example, contained the following services:

- Answers to over 400 common queries
- An Instant Library of over 300 articles
- A Getting Help list of available support services

- Personal Stories depicting how people coped with their disease
- Ask an Expert replies to specific questions
- A Discussion Group as an ongoing forum among users
- Assessment for self-appraisal
- Decision Aid to help consider options
- Action Plan to guide the implementation of decisions
- Health Charts, a diary for monitoring progress
- A large glossary of relevant terms. (Gustafson et al. 1993)

Support at Home

Because at least half of all adults will at some point become caregivers to an aging parent, spouse, sibling, or friend, home caregivers will increasingly provide a valuable form of health care that cannot be replaced by outside caregivers. Yet they experience more mental and physical health problems and bear more social isolation than other Americans. More than half of those who care for demented elders suffer depression (Monk 1988).

IT support at home for these caregivers and for people with home-confining conditions can become a new form of useful and supportive information, education, and communication. One program, for example, uses a computer-automated telephone outreach system to routinely assess the needs of chemotherapy outpatients, such as transportation to the hospital and assistance with activities of daily living. It also reminds them to take medications and keep appointments and follows up immediately after discharge from the hospital to ensure that they receive planned services (Christ and Siegel 1990; Monk 1988).

Using IT support, physical health care data can be collected through computer terminals in patients' homes or in senior centers, replacing time-consuming phone calls or trips to the doctor's office. In one demonstration in England, women with high-risk pregnancies living in a rural community were able to periodically monitor their fetus with an electronic device used with a telephone link, thus avoiding a costly, time-consuming overnight trip to a hospital (Gott 1993).

Computerized personal emergency response systems for distance monitoring of elders and other special groups in the United States allow them more independence (Rice 1987). In a program at one rehabilitation center, a video telephone was used to communicate regularly with elders who, should they have a home accident or have difficulty obtaining food during bad weather, could receive immediate service around the clock. This supported a much more satisfying quality of life for elders living alone at a much lower cost than being an inpatient (Gott 1993).

A Missing Piece

What is missing from these glimpses of the possibilities for using information technology in the delivery of health services are scenarios that depict an electronic web of health agencies and other community-based organizations, the ones that continue to offer broader health support over more sustained timespans than medical providers are able to do because of the limits of their medical tools and the limits of their budgets. The case study that follows suggests the prospects as well as the difficulties of embedding IT in the ongoing support structure of community life.

References

Agency for Health Care Policy Research (AHCPR). 1992a. *Evaluation of a Comprehensive Hospital Information System*. Washington, DC: DHHS.

———. 1992b. *Proceedings of the Annual Symposium on Computer Applications in Medical Care*. Washington, DC: DHHS.

Aird, J. 1992. "The Missing Link." *Health Service Journal* (June): 28–29.

Anderson, M. 1988. "Evaluation of a Microcomputer-Enhanced Intervention of Elementary School Children." *Family & Community Health* 1: 36–47.

Association of North Carolina Boards of Health. 1991. ANCBH Health Leadership Institute Annual Report. Raleigh, NC.

Barker, K., E. Allan, and E. S. Swensson. 1989. "Effect of Technological Changes in Information Transfer on the Delivery of Pharmacy Services." *American Journal of Pharmaceutical Education* Winter: 53.

Bliss, G., L. Foster, and K. Ho. 1991. "Mapping Community Health Information." Unpublished Report. Victoria, B.C.: British Columbia Ministry of Health.

Brennan, P., and J. Fitzpatrick. 1993. "On the Essential Integration of Nursing and Informatics." *Nursing Informatics* (November): 797–803.

Chan, L., and N. Schonfeld. 1992. *How Much Is Lost During Information Processing: A Case Study of Pediatric Emergency Room Records*. Paper presented at the 120th Annual Meeting of the American Public Health Association, Washington, DC, November.

Christ, G., and K. Siegel. 1990. "Monitoring Quality of Life Needs of Cancer Patients." *Cancer* 65: 760–65.

Commonwealth Department of Health. 1992. *The Future of General Practice*. National Health Strategy Issues Paper No. 3. Canberra, A.C.T., Australia, 147–58.

Couto, R. 1986. *Apples and Health Care*. Nashville, TN: Vanderbilt University.

Detmer, D., and E. Steen. 1993. "Patient Records in the Information Age." *Issues in Science and Technology* (Spring): 36–39.

Ellis, L. 1987. "Computer-Based Patient Education." *Computers in Human Services* 2 (3–4): 117–30.

Evans, R., et al. 1993. "Development of an Automated Antibiotic Consultant." *MD Computing* 10: 17–22.

Friede, A., J. Reid, and H. Ory. 1993. "CDC WONDER: A Comprehensive On-line Public Health Information System of the Centers for Disease Control and Prevention." *American Journal of Public Health* 83 (9): 1289–94.

General Accounting Office. 1993. *Automated Medical Records*. Washington, DC: U.S. Congress, 30 April.

Gogdetz, A. 1985. "Good Medical Care in Nursing Homes." *American Journal of Public Health* 75 (3): 277–80.

Gott, M. 1993. "Telehealth and Telemedicine in the Electronic Home." Unpublished Report. European Foundation for the Improvement of Living and Working Conditions, Dublin.

Grundner, T.M., and R. E. Garrett. 1986. "Interactive Medical Telecomputing: An Alternative Approach to Community Health Education." *New England Journal of Medicine* 314 (15): 1866–68.

Gustafson, D., et al. 1993. "A Computer-Based System for Empowering Persons Living with AIDS/HIV Infection through Education and Social Support." *Interactive Healthcare News* (3): 1.

Harris Consulting Group. 1994. "Preliminary Study: Consumer Demand for Health Information." Unpublished Report. Washington, DC.

Harrison, M., and B. Green. 1986."Computers in Health Visiting." *Midwife-Health Visitor-Community Nursing (UK)* 22 (4): 110–14.

Hekelman, F., S. Niles, and P. Brennan. 1993. "Gerontological Home Care: A Prescription for Distance Continuing Education." *Computers in Nursing*.

Hodge, T. D., and M. N. Steele. 1991. "Alberta Health Units' Information Technology Strategic Plan." Unpublished Report. Edmonton, Alberta: Public Health Division, Alberta Health.

Institute of Medicine. 1991. *The Computer-Based Patient Record. An Essential Technology for Health Care*. Washington, DC: National Academy Press.

International Medical Benefits and Risk Foundation. 1993. *Report on Patient Information*. Washington, DC: IMBRF.

Klein, E. 1993. "Automating Home Care." *Healthcare Informatics* (August): 22–27.

Kosidlak, J., and K. Kerpelman. 1987. "Managing Community Health Nursing: APC Tool for Assessing, Monitoring and Planning the Distribution of Public Health Nursing Resources at the Community Level." *Computers in Nursing* 5 (5): 175–80.

McDonald, S., and W. Tierney. 1992. "Effects of Computer Reminders for Influenza Vaccination on Morbidity During Influenza Epidemics." *MD Computing* 9 (5): 304–12.

Monk, A. 1988. "Aging, Loneliness, and Communications." *American Behavioral Scientist* 31 (5): 532–60.

Nath, L. M., and K. Tuli. 1991. *A Computer Based System for Community Health Care in Rural North India*. Centre for Community Medicine. All India Institute of Medical Science, New Delhi, June.

National Center for Nursing Research. 1993. *Nursing Informatics: Enhancing Patient Care*. Bethesda, MD: National Institutes of Health.

Office of Technology Assessment (OTA). 1993. *Protecting Privacy in Computerized Medical Information*. Washington, DC: U.S. Congress, October.

Omnibus Budget Reconciliation Act of 1990. 1990. Conference Report to Accompany H.R. 5835. Report 101-964, p. 162. Washington, DC: U.S. Government Printing Office, 27 October.

"Overview of Health Care." 1993. *Smart Card News* 2: 10.

Pangalos, G. 1992. "Design and Implementation of Computer-readable Patient Data Cards." *Medical Informatics* 17 (4): 243–56.

Paperny, D. M., and J. R. Starn. 1989. "Adolescent Pregnancy Prevention by Health Education Computer Games: Computer-Assisted Instruction of Knowledge and Attitudes." *Pediatrics* 83: 742–52.

Paperny, D. M., J. Y. Aono, R. M. Lehman, S. L. Hammar, and J. Risser. 1990. "Computer-Assisted Detection and Intervention in Adolescent High-risk Health Behaviors." *The Journal of Pediatrics* 116 (March): 456–62.

Petryshen, P., and G. Pelekis. 1992. "Multimedia Applications in Nursing for Computer-Based Staff Training and Patient Education." *Journal of Continuing Education* (3): 23.

Physician Computer Network, Inc. 1992. *Annual Report.* Laurence Harbor, NJ.

Public Health Service. 1993. *Community Services Network Project Summary.* Washington, DC: DHHS, August.

Ramirez, S. A. 1991. *Are There World-Wide Applications for a Computer-Based System Designed to Provide Linkages Between a Health Sciences Center and Remote or Rural Health Care Providers and Health Care Recipients?* Texas Tech University Health Sciences Center, School of Nursing, Lubbock, TX.

Reichard, J. 1993. "Health Industry Wields Computers in Cost Quality Battle." *Medicine & Health Perspectives* 22 March: 1–4.

Rice, M. 1987. *Toward Harnessing New Electronic Technologies to Meet the Needs of Elderly People.* Aspen Forum Report #4. Aspen Institute, New York.

Robinson, T., and P. Walters. 1987. "Changing Community Health Behaviors with a Health Promotion Computer Network." In *Proceedings: Computer Applications in Medical Care,* edited by W. Stead. Washington, DC: IEEE.

Scheske, C. 1991. *Long Term Strategic Directions in Health Care Communications.* Health Care Services Division, Co-operators Data Services Ltd., Regina, Saskatchewan.

Schneider, S. 1986. "Trial of an Online Behavioral Smoking Cessation Program." *Computers and Human Behavior* 2 (4): 277–86.

"Technology Payoff." 1993. *Business Week,* 14 June: 57–79.

Thomas, R., J. Cahill, and R. Durlak. 1993. "Health Education for Teens Using Mobile Information Technology." Unpublished Report. Albany: New York State Department of Health.

U.S. Congress. 1992. *Redefining AIDS: Its Impact on Health and Disability Entitlement Spending.* House Committee on the Budget. Republican Staff Report. Washington, DC.

Wright, C. 1985. "Computer-Aided Nursing Diagnosis for Community Health Nurses." *Nursing Clinics of North America* 29 (3): 487–95.

CHAPTER

6

SUPPORTING HOME CAREGIVERS IN INDY

Community Information Networks to Homes and among Homes

HOW CAN postindustrial diseases like Alzheimer's and AIDS be borne humanely by those who succumb and by their intimates? How do colleges that educate nurses, historically the handmaidens of medical doctors, find collegial equity in universities and in the emerging health care system, where services are delivered outside institutional walls and costs and access are primary issues? These questions seemed to come together in a project about a new way to help home caregivers use information technology in Indy.

The Local Scene

Indy is an important city because it is so ordinary, so typical of many northcentral urban areas—middle size, losing its population base; blue collar, losing its manufacturing base. In the early nineties, its families were more likely than the rest of the state to be headed by women, to be unemployed, and to be poor. Yet the mayor and city council had attempted to invest in community and infrastructure developments such as housing and sanitation, within the limits of revenues, deficits, and fiscal competition from health care costs and police protection (Bureau of the Census 1988; APHA 1992).

In spite of its problems, Indy had some priceless assets. It had a tradition of home ownership and a history of community—the capacity for groups to work together for some common good—attested to by longtime community support for its recognized cultural, educational, and medical institutions. The contrast between past and present could be used either as a source of inspiration to create a hopeful future or as a forecast of a downward spiral for Indy.

A Freenet

One, but only one, set of tools to help strengthen community life today, to develop a human infrastructure for promoting economic and social development as the ground for health and well-being, is community information technology. Indy's computer network, a freenet, was open to any user without charge. Dozens of freenets were spreading to cities across the country, sponsored by universities, libraries, and other nonprofit coalitions, members of the fledgling National Public Telecomputing Network. Freenet, with its electronic community bulletin board, promoted the discussion of election issues in the nineties by posting position statements from candidates in all parties. This was one of its aims—the beginnings of "teledemocracy"—using community computers linked to telecommunications to disseminate information about city, state, and national government to the electorate (National Public Telecomputing Network 1993).

Proponents of freenet believed that local advocacy for community issues across an electronic net could help mobilize people and support collaborative action—for those who could access the system. The accessibility problem became evident on the Indy freenet soon after it began. It was first designed for educational purposes. Very soon, the public entered the computer system and it was transformed into a public service to answer the public's questions.

By the early 1990s there were over 40,000 people logging into the system over 10,000 times a day. This kind of momentum was evident across the country. Many in this computer-literate vanguard subscribed to the philosophical position of the National Public Telecomputing Network:

> . . . whether we are going to live in an Information Age is no longer at issue. We are. The only question which remains is what we are going to do about it—whether we, as a society, will be able to use this new technology to more effectively (in the words of James Madison) " . . . arm ourselves with the power which knowledge gives." (NPTN 1993)

The movement-like quality of this vanguard would grow toward its goal of a nation-linking and world-linking electronic network open to all who could use a telephone and a computer terminal. Meanwhile, what of the vast majority who had no access to community IT?

This was the question raised by others in Indy, and they attempted to find ways to answer it.

An Agency Net

The very existence of freenet made possible the development of other forms of community IT that could widen the circle of potential users beyond advantaged individuals. The net meant that groups and organizations—if they had the necessary expertise and hardware—could multiply, extend, and improve the services they offered people in the community. One of Indy's oldest health and welfare agencies attempted to use this electronic toolbox to evaluate and improve its community services.

In the late eighties, the Indy Elder Welfare Institute began an interagency database among its five collaborating agencies in several counties to assess how effective their programs were in providing respite service to home caregivers of people with Alzheimer's Disease. During the first year of operation, they received about one telephone inquiry a day about the respite service, which provided temporary in-home care or day care for the patient. Having recorded the callers' queries in the computer system, their analysis showed that they were not reaching all of the people who needed their service because their fees were not affordable, especially for low-income families.

The computerized system worked effectively; the evaluation of the data was useful; but the project failed. Most of the sister agencies dropped the system, and even the Elder Institute did not incorporate the system into its own in-house computer system. The main reasons were organizational ones: under tight budgets, there were no incentives to continue, no imperatives, no costly supporting expertise to solve technical problems, customize software, train new staff, or manage the system. In a word, no funds.

Without these supports, the qualms voiced by social workers about "depersonalizing" their contacts with clients and feeling "the machine" might take over making clinical decisions—in effect, making them less central and essential—would be a strong deterrent to using IT. Nonetheless, the exercise became a backdrop, a fund of experience within the institute to provide consultative support for an innovation in community IT that was soon to begin at the university's college of nursing.

Demands for Innovation

The new information technologies were being accepted in health services, but with serious questions: would IT dehumanize an already often impersonal and remote system? Would it displace the interpersonal rapport that not only social case workers but also nurses and others attempt to establish with their patients? Would it displace some health and social service professionals?

In any case, the imperatives of controlling rising health care costs, the growing numbers of chronically ill, disabled, and frail people of all ages, the increase in single person and single parent households, and the widening scope of high-powered, low-cost IT virtually mandated continuous efforts to use these tools in the service of health care. But the question continued to be how to find humane and acceptable ways to do it. How can IT augment, eliminate, or find substitutes for some face-to-face encounters between people with health problems and the formal health care delivery system?

Half of adult Americans will serve as caregivers to an aging parent, spouse, brother, sister, or friend; and growing numbers of patients are being treated outside hospitals. So, caregivers themselves will need at least as much support at home as the people who are ill. At the same time, the cost of services will have to be minimized. Yet, in the 1980s, the evaluation of home care technologies was limited to advanced therapies such as ventilators and hyperalimentation systems, virtually neglecting information technology (OTA 1984, 1990).

The typical ways to support caregivers and home care patients included social support groups and personal contact with professional caregivers. But the benefits of support groups, as well as other face-to-face services such as counseling and education, were often not accessible. Attendance at meetings required physical energy, willingness to associate with the stigmatized and the dying, and sometimes the additional burden of finding someone to stay with the patient. Contact with professionals was costly, sometimes not available, and frequently did not provide answers to the everyday problems of living with an ill family member (OTA 1990).

The actual cost of caring for a progressively demented elder at home, for example, was almost $20,000 a year, excluding the costs of informal services (about $1,500 in the mid-nineties). Most of the overall costs were paid out-of-pocket by families. Those who could not afford the expenses were more likely to do without than to obtain public support. The irony was that a large share of the costs were for support not of the patient, but of the home caregiver—for services such as in-home companion and adult day care services (Weinberger et al. 1993). Nationally, the cost of nursing home and home care for Alzheimer's was about $90 billion a year. The Alzheimer's caregivers in Indy who became participants in the community IT innovation called CareNet had themselves used three different health or social services in the month before the project began.

The need for such support was further revealed as caregivers experienced more physical and mental health problems and were less able to participate in ordinary social life than other people. Up to half or more caregivers of demented elders, for example, experienced depression. Depression was especially severe among women, who make up the vast majority of caregivers (OTA 1990).

Other people with the kinds of health conditions that require some form of in-home support were mothers with new or premature babies, parents with chronically ill children, people living with AIDS and their partners, one-day surgery patients, and those in rural areas.

Parent of Innovation

Awareness of these health and health care delivery issues, of Indy's wide-reaching freenet, and of the variety of IT innovations germinating in the city permeated the leadership of the university's college of nursing in the early eighties. The school began a highly successful capital campaign, the development of new educational programs and research projects, and a concerted and constant effort to become a responsive part of the Indy community of organizations. An initial gift of $100,000 from local corporate leaders as a discretionary fund was a distinct incentive for an outward focus for the college. This outward thrust gave the college the unusual status of having a budget surplus in the early nineties, which it proudly displayed in its annual report.

Just as community contacts and projects improved the college's prospects for acquiring large gifts, its aggressive and successful search for research grant meant prestige and a stronger voice in campus politics.

To bring the tradition of nursing into the world of the information age, it was the school's view that, in the words of the dean,

> Nursing is fundamentally an information processing discipline. . . . Nurses make observations about patients, convert these data elements to information using nursing judgments, take action premised on the available information, and then store it. . . . Nursing cannot meet its social mandate without informatics technologies.

Support for Innovation

> Some administrators like to hire famous people.
> I like to hire people who *want* to be famous.

These words from the dean were echoed in the college's support of energetic, fame-seeking new faculty it built up its development office to help frame proposals and seek appropriate funders. It allowed time for proposal development and allocated funds to hire student help for faculty and pay for travel to negotiate with potential funders.

This was the climate into which this private college of nursing recruited nurses with IT interests who could "do it better than anyone"—that is, they could develop IT innovations in the community for improving nursing practice, evaluate them, obtain external funds, and in the process strengthen the status of the college.

With this kind of backing, the new recruits began an innovative niche for the college. The work paid off in large grant funds from public and private sources, and new courses, research programs, community linkages.

Developing the Idea

The initial thinking about computers in this period of computer-infancy in campus life of the mid-eighties emphasized its rational potential. It was not a belief in the omniscience of the machine, not a faith in artificial intelligence, but the view of a few nurse IT-innovators that

> computer-based decision aids . . . can help people better understand the problems they face by clarifying the options available, the values and criteria for selection among options, and the uncertainties involved in selection, as well as helping in the final selection.

The impetus to think in broader terms came from the imperatives of the college's community-dependent developmental focus and the research pressures on the faculty novitiate. Having discussed the freenet through scattered professional contacts, the network's technical possibilities became the topic of ongoing informal discussions with campus freenet proponents. The college had a proposal for developing a home interactive computer system, but it was admittedly not well-developed and was turned down as a "crazy idea" by one large foundation. There seemed to be little computer awareness in nurse-funding organizations at the time. Thus, freenet, with its IT expertise and ties to sociology and psychology, became the nurturing womb for CareNet. Discussions at the university's Alzheimer's center initiated the idea of using home-based computers to support Alzheimer's caregivers—the center had just begun developing a general public information service on freenet for people interested in the disease.

Finding Funds

Ideas are easy and fun. The hard job, the months of effort it takes to write a fundable proposal, fell to the college of nursing, which completed the task in the fall of 1987. The college provided its IT-innovators with graduate student assistance and contacts in the federal funding network. The federal contacts were known to say "I can't advise you, but if I *could*, I would say you should. . . ." After "massive rewriting," another variation of the proposal was submitted where the "new money" was: AIDS research. The project was reconceived as self-care nursing for AIDS to justify its funding.

To obtain funds for testing CareNet, the AIDS and Alzheimer's grant-writing teams, whose academic careers could be enhanced by involvement in a funded research project, conformed the design of their proposals to current National Institutes of Health research priorities. These included investigations in specific disease processes, the use of technology (defined as computers to deliver self-care nursing services), and strategies to reduce the ill effects on home caregivers. These priorities were driven by both the search for cost savings and technology developments.

The strategy to obtain funds was to seek several sources and define the problem and its importance in terms of the agenda, priorities, and interests of the specific funding source. To potential nurse funders, for example, the proposal emphasized nurse-related components, pointing out that computer technology might be "a very effective medium for extending nursing services beyond traditional caregiving situations. Currently many persons cannot obtain needed nursing services" (because of lack of insurance, too few nurses in rural areas, and too many patients demanding care). Nonetheless, the proposal assured the funder that CareNet would "extend and augment, not replace, direct nursing care."

The team also stated that "nursing service delivered or augmented by a computer network has never been tested." Studies had shown only that nurses could use computers to resolve work-related decisions and that the delivery of rural nursing care could be more efficient through the use of computer networks. CareNet, however, would provide a way for all users to share self-care knowledge, thus expanding "understanding of how nursing care can be modified to include computer mediated nursing care."

They also framed the specific needs of AIDS patients within what they knew to be high-profile issues among nurse leaders and funders—namely, access to services, improving self-care and prevention, and getting acknowledgment for advanced clinical services roles for nurses. The team argued that many persons with AIDS, because of insurance gaps or their desire to remain anonymous, remain outside the formal health care system until late stages of the disease. Earlier contact with professional nurses might promote self-care and forestall some of the preventable complications of AIDS. Such people, because of the complexity of their condition, should have the informal advice they obtain from each other overseen and supervised by a nurse. For this purpose, the team proposed an electronic service providing an expert AIDS nurse to review messages daily and respond where necessary with accurate information.

The rationale was that a longtime nursing role was to provide support to patients and their informal caregivers as they cope with the problems associated with home-based care, and this was consistent with "nurses' information broker role." It would improve self-care, but because home care also increased demands on staff nurses for monitoring care and traveling to an ever-growing number of clients, a new set of supportive techniques was necessary.

The CareNet System

The software for the proposed CareNet network had a decision module, an electronic communication pathway, and a database specifically designed to improve caregivers' knowledge and problem-solving capacity. These were to increase their social and professional contacts, and give them access to necessary information 24 hours a day. Because it gave people access to other caregivers and to health professionals, the system was hoped to "normalize" the illness experience rather than "medicalize" it, answering questions that commonly occur and providing anonymity to encourage patients and caregivers to ask questions.

The daily use of CareNet was to be overseen by a project nurse who was both a group facilitator and a clinical expert. As facilitator, she or he monitored public communication and individual participation, then placed messages on the bulletin board designed to encourage responses from others, building a kind of "support group without walls." A third task was that of a systems operator—or in the jargon of IT, a "sysop," a person who maintains the program with updates, answers questions about its operations, and generally troubleshoots problems for users when the system does not work to their satisfaction.

In effect, the project teams proposed a marriage between information technology and the new and growing needs in health services, hoping to produce a new form of community-focused IT, a new set of tools for the future. This technology was not claimed as a perfect solution, nor a complete one. The team acknowledged that computer-mediated communication was both more and less rich than face-to-face exchange. The nuances of feeling were missing, and so was some of the meaning of words. There was both more anonymity and more flexibility in when and how to use it. People could identify themselves with self-selected code names in place of their own names. They could use their own time frame as well. The uniqueness of CareNet was that it sought to deliver clinical services, including individualized counseling and guidance, in the home, and to do so with people who were "computer naive," having never had a computer of their own.

The AIDS project was eventually funded at $600,000 for three years by the National Center for Nursing Research at the National Institutes of Health. The Alzheimer's proposal, once approved, was passed through the federal bureaucracy in search of available funds, traveling from the National Center for Health Services Research to NIH and eventually to the National Institute on Aging. It was finally funded for two years. Its $750,000 was designated for a randomized field evaluation of a novel computer network. Both projects were known as CareNet.

Project Organization

Much of 1987 and 1988 had been spent juggling grant writing and rewriting, guessing at whether and when the proposals would be approved and funded, putting together project teams, and in the process, plying the web of contacts with the groups and organizations that were essential for successful development of the projects. Perhaps because of the greater political currency and visibility of AIDS at the national level, its funds moved more quickly through the pipeline and were first to arrive for the first attempt at CareNet.

The project teams each had a director to coordinate the 10 or 12 people involved, and each team had varied backgrounds and career agendas. Each director had different time commitments, but basically believed that to some degree the project would enhance their careers, as an extraordinary research opportunity, as a vehicle for generating publications, as supplemental income during graduate education, as evidence of their academic "ownership" of a new idea, and other prestigious "halo effects" from the studies.

In the college as a whole, the CareNet concept and that of IT generally was so new that it was not a reality in the minds of the faculty. The teams may have felt that they were working in a kind of future time warp.

In order to work effectively, they had to to arrive at a common understanding about purposes and procedures. For example, since most of the members were nurses, they were faced with an entirely new context for determining what a "nursing intervention" meant when it did not occur in the customary face-to-face situation, and when the timing of the clinician's response was no longer seconds but could be hours or days. The questions that arose included many that required new organizational decisions in the face of new technology:

- Should the moderator's response take an individual therapeutic approach or a group support approach (e.g., by encouraging others on the network to respond first)? (The group approach predominated.)
- Do the users *want* therapy?
- Do the moderator and the trainer who sets up the equipment at homes have to be nurses?
- Should electronic personal attacks be allowed and inaccurate or other messages be removed? (None were removed, but attacks and inaccuracies did not pass without a response.)

In time, CareNet users became very comfortable with each other, and even those who had electronically uttered racist epithets unwittingly became CareNet friends with others of different races, unimpeded by racial stereotypes.

After all the discussions, writing, and planning, at the time of the initial pilot studies, the team thinking and the stated rationale were that CareNet's main aim and value was to help solve the frustration and agonies of caregivers' uncertainties about their chronically ill loved ones. This perspective or professional bias, among others, would change.

Organizational Linkages

More important than melding the teams' varied personal agendas into a common effort was the larger reality that demanded cooperation with organizations essential to the projects. The agendas, priorities, and resource commitments of these collaborators were sometimes very different from CareNet's.

The overarching resource for CareNet was the citywide electronic network, freenet. While in principle the college could establish a special system linking CareNet to each home-based terminal, the existence of freenet and its technical support was not only a convenience, but also a way of literally connecting the college to the entire campus, the IT administration in particular, and the Indy community. This could serve the longer-term goals of the college and CareNet's future as well.

CareNet in a Nonorganized Environment: People Living with AIDS

In the mid-1980s, with AIDS linked to gays in the public mind, and gays in Indy fearing discrimination, there was little visible, organizational infrastructure through which CareNet could reach the homosexuals among its clientele. There was even less structure for reaching intravenous drug users and other groups at high risk for AIDS. This relatively nonorganized environment meant that the CareNet team had to look for volunteer participants through its most familiar and ready source, the university's medical center clinic, which served over 800 HIV-infected patients.

The medical center was undergoing a large expansion and reorganization program, repositioning itself in the health care market. It used tactics such as a television advertising campaign, "Shaping the Future of Medicine," to explain to consumers its "breadth of services, expertise, and research intensity," because market research showed that Indy citizens perceived its character as an aloof institution. Cooperation with

CareNet would be consistent with the medical center's interest in having community-oriented services that were easily understood and approved by the public. The medical center was dependent on Indy citizens for both the expansion of its services and the patient-based experience needed by the health professionals in its educational and research programs.

Hurdling the Professions

The groundwork for CareNet at the medical clinic was first laid by getting the support of a physician who was a single mother, a specialist whose interest was in the then out-of-the-mainstream issue of preventing AIDS in teens. "After all," she was known to say, "I'm going to have one someday." The CareNet team then obtained permission from the chief physician.

This next step was a more difficult task. The chief physician had to be assured that CareNet was not intended to replace physicians and that the project would be explained to his clinic staff to obtain their voluntary agreement to help recruit participants. He said he worried that CareNet would offer too much information, confusing people or encouraging them to think they knew enough to take care of themselves. Or it would promote "nontraditional medicine" and "legitimize trash" by encouraging users to advise each other to try home remedies or other treatments. To this the project's answer was to have a specialist nurse monitor all public communications and use physician expertise for any questionable issues.

In short order, the clinic medical staff was fully briefed, their questions answered, and assurances given that the project would not require any clinic resources apart from space to interview one patient at a time. The clinic itself had its own AIDS research grant from the National Institutes of Health, and so was compatible in principle with CareNet.

The AIDS team manager was a uniquely qualified nurse, self-described as "culturally compatible" with many AIDS participants because of his sex and sexual preference. Through his contact with the then low-visibility gay community, he was helping to set up a center for gays with HIV infection, the Homeplace. However, even he had to learn to develop a more inviting, less "professional" style if he was to obtain patients' cooperation. When he began to wear casual clothes, as opposed to a business suit, he became more successful with the patients.

These and other insights were part of the training of the CareNet staff, along with sensitivities and precautions about making home visits in Indy's inner city. The team had several unanticipated experiences. One young single mother, HIV-infected and addicted to crack cocaine, lived "in squalor at a crack house" in a room with her four young children. In such a chaotic environment, the least of the problems was to find adequate wiring and space to install CareNet equipment. Yet, the IT system was set up, and in time this new user linked up with another woman, moved out, and got "clean" with the help of the AIDS clinic. She seemed to use her CareNet as a healthy substitute when she felt the need for a "fix." Another woman used CareNet as her main contact with the outside world while she hid from her husband when he was released from prison.

Such episodes shattered stereotypes of home computer users and were one extreme on the long spectrum of individuals' patterns of IT use that challenged the CareNet project in its implementation and aftermath. A more expected challenge was obtaining the expert assistance of the university's office of technology, which managed freenet. CareNet was able to get the support it needed mainly because its funds would be used to support its linkage to freenet and related technical assistance.

As a day-to-day matter for the team, the issue with freenet was how to get the "techies" to realize "they could help human beings out there." The way to do it, they found, was to make the project human, with the stories about crack houses and fearful wives rather than with research data.

The lesson learned for reaching hard-to-reach people and for dealing with CareNet users themselves was to "make the hardware sensitive and caring by providing people support," by offering someone to help each person enter the electronic group—in effect, to get people hooked after getting them linked.

The AIDS project began with a feasibility period of several months during which the team learned basic ways to approach their clientele.

Developing the Software

The information component of the computer program was a kind of AIDS encyclopedia. But tailoring it to its audience required in-depth contact with the prospective users to learn what they wanted to know and how best to package it. By interviewing people living with AIDS for several months and visiting the homes of infected gays and intravenous drug users and their sex partners, the team was able to enrich the encyclopedia with familiar idioms that improved its usefulness.

The nurses also learned what contacts people with AIDS were and were not using, and why. Support groups and clinicians were the primary resources available to HIV-infected persons, yet almost half said they were reluctant to attend support groups because they found the experience upsetting, depressing, and focused on illness. They were also concerned about anonymity and the availability of transportation.

One unanticipated effect of this preparatory period was the strengthened credibility of the project in the gay community. Another was favorable publicity for the college of nursing, as the project realized that "the marquee is the key," that is, the public face of the project was crucial to its acceptance by the community; public relations was important.

Having gathered the information they needed, the team organized it into common themes, with key words for each section of the electronic encyclopedia. There was factual information about AIDS ("What Is AIDS?") and clinical information ("When to Call a Doctor"). The database gave announcements of local services ("Where Can I Find a Support Group?"). Information within each title was prioritized so that the most important was explained first. Text was designed for a sixth grade reading level.

Another component of the computer program, the public and private messaging system, offered private mail and a public bulletin board moderated by a nurse. She or he used specific group techniques in deciding how to respond to the messages of CareNet users, such as support, information giving, silence, encouraging expression of feelings and ideas, acceptance, reassurance, clarification, and interpretation. The moderator would use public postings to point out themes to the group in a very directive manner, or to ask group members to comment and offer suggestions. These nurse moderators reviewed each message within 24 hours of its posting and acknowledged them all. In this way, in addition to the traditional one-to-one relationship between patient and practitioner, a one-to-many relationship was always present.

In addition to the information and communications components, the third element was a module for decision modeling. It emphasized drawing out from the decision maker his or her own understanding of the problem and the alternatives open to solving the problem. This was to lead the user to redefine the problem, increasing the clarity of her or his preferences and thereby improving self-care from the caregiver's point of view.

The question of incurring legal liabilities for giving advice and other professional health services over the network had to be addressed. This had been readily handled by freenet, where disclaimers appeared each time the network was accessed. In places where professional advice was provided, the professional's name was identified (in the case of CareNet, this was the nurse clinician) along with advice to users to discuss issues with their own clinician.

Hardware

The choice of hardware for CareNet was based on criteria that would make it a doable program for the future. This meant that the equipment had to be inexpensive (no more than the current price of a television set at $350), simple to use and maintain, durable, and "not very sexy." It would have to be a "plain vanilla" model that would not tempt users to try to sell it. Another issue was availability of suppliers. One computer giant was willing to give CareNet a good price for a complicated laptop that it was having a hard time selling on the open market. A lesser known firm, having become interested in the concept and recognizing the advertising and public relations value of its cooperation, arranged a better price for its terminals and modems for CareNet and so was chosen as the supplier.

CareNet equipment consisted of a computer terminal, a keyboard, and a modem connecting the terminal to the telephone. Each caregiver was initially provided with the system in their home, and later loaned it for indefinite use. Participants had access to CareNet through a personal code. At the request of AIDS clients' partners who wanted to use the system, they too received access codes. Each user was trained in his or her own home by a project nurse during a session lasting about an hour and a half.

Testing CareNet

After the pilot trial, the CareNet team moved into the main evaluation phase of the project. It used two groups in a one-year field experiment. Computers were installed in the homes of 27 randomly selected persons living with AIDS, while another comparison group of 26 similar people was given other information and support resources, but not the electronic system. Participants in both groups received a self-care guidebook published by the project team. This was a diary with one page for each week of the study to record users' health care contacts. Project nurses made telephone calls to participants to allow them to describe what they had done in the previous week. These individuals were reimbursed $15 per month for their participation, and payment was released after each telephone contact was made (for a total of $160 on average for the 12-month period).

To some users, the end of the project was like "taking away a pill that worked," even though there would continue to be an open discussion area on AIDS that AIDS CareNet users could continue to access on Indy's freenet. In an organizational sense, however, the project had made no plans to continue CareNet's unique services, since it was experimental and therefore there was no way of knowing whether it would work. The project did not seek funds for ongoing operations. The formal intention was to simply offer the software—minus the question-answer, nurse-moderated service—to freenet.

But the project manager attempted a more organized type of "technology transfer" by offering CareNet to the gays' Homeplace facility and training the minuscule Homeplace staff to use it. Without further back-up, however, it was effectively dismantled by a new Homeplace manager who believed that gays ought to meet face-to-face, preferably at Homeplace. Another informal effort to provide the question-answer service, run by a graduate student nurse at the college, also faded after a short while when the student went on to other things. Thus, without pre-program planning for the technology transfer to another organization, even successful community IT was not sustainable.

But CareNet was better prepared and had better prospects for the long term in the more organized community environment of Alzheimer's patients.

CareNet in an Organized Environment: Alzheimer's Caregivers

Alzheimer's Disease had been in the public mind for a somewhat longer time than AIDS, and was also better accepted and less stigmatized in the 1980s. Along with widening public and private support, there developed a formal organizational infrastructure for research, treatment, education, and family services. This was the organizational network that CareNet had to tap. The prime players in Indy were the university medical center's Alzheimer's Center, which had federal funds for research, treatment, and training. The other was the local Alzheimer's Association, a nonprofit group that offered support services to families and that was financed mainly by members' dues.

Collaboration and Competition

CareNet's tie to the Alzheimer's Center, which was essential for recruiting families for participation in the project, was a relationship that was effectively maintained, but only gingerly. The problems grew out of the mutual dependence and semicompatibility of the two units.

The Background

The evolution of CareNet was the backdrop to this smoldering conflict. The first CareNet grant application was submitted to federal funders in the fall of 1987, after several months of preparation. Earlier concept papers had served as trial balloons to other potential funders earlier in the year. The idea was developed more fully during 1987 and 1988, when brainstorming was going on among freenet proponents, the CareNet team, and the university's Alzheimer's Center.

The center began to support the development of its own form of a computer-based Alzheimer's information system, to be programmed for freenet users and known as AlzCenter. The center's core funding came from an NIH grant that required it to have an education and information transfer component for the public, its patients, and professionals. AlzCenter was to serve that purpose.

AlzCenter was described as a "computer-based system designed to address some of the limitations of currently available information and support activities for caregivers of persons with Alzheimer's." It consisted of question-answer modules, to be serviced by professionals from the center; an information section listing support group meetings and printed and other resources; and bulletin boards for the general public to discuss related issues, as well as one for caregivers. These were monitored by volunteer staff of the local Alzheimer's Association chapter. The program was announced to freenet users in May of 1990 after several weeks of testing.

As described by one of the initial groups involved in its development, AlzCenter followed a "medical model," attempting primarily to offer professional advice on request, and "passively" making up-to-date information available by an electronic route. Since typical freenet users were in their mid-twenties—older people tended to have neither interest in nor access to computers—AlzCenter was used very little; perhaps three people prior to mid-1991 posted up to 300 messages in the first 11 months. Questions were in fact "seeded" into the system by the center to try to stimulate interest. The underlying aim of the effort, however, was to use it as a "tantalizer" for prospective funders, in hopes of obtaining an adequate staffing arrangement.

CareNet's request to the Alzheimer's Center to have access to the families of its patients for their prospective participation in the CareNet trial was, in the eyes of some at the center, "a fresh wind over a dormant seed"—the possibility, "the chutzpah, organization, and finances" to make the AlzCenter idea work. Yet the inherent conflict among the brainstorming designers was soon to surface.

CareNet, first funded for AIDS in 1988 and begun for Alzheimer's caregivers in 1989, operated on-line from May of 1990 to June of 1991. It was self-described—and contrasted from AlzCenter—as following a self-help/social support model for "computer-naive" people, in particular those who were thought to be hard to reach or "unteachable." Users were to be transformed from mere readers of information to interactors with a clinical specialist nurse and with each other, and were expected to find answers to questions that "only caregivers who were living through the same experiences could know." This was to encourage a "fact and affect-based" system made easier by creating a highly simplified and transparent technology at a time when graphical software was not typical.

The Conflict

Both AlzCenter and CareNet were ready to go on-line in the spring of 1990. Yet, if CareNet families used CareNet on the freenet, they could also access AlzCenter with its similar types of information and could "contaminate" CareNet's research. A second issue emerged when CareNet concepts and language were suspected of being used but not acknowledged in the Alzheimer's Center's renewal application for its federal grant funding of the AlzCenter system. Here then were conflicts about the systems' operations and control and who owned what ideas and concepts.

It was in the interests of both sides to resolve the issues so that each could proceed unimpeded. It would not do to have two entities continue their grievances and mar the larger relations between their parent organizations, namely, the colleges of nursing and of medicine.

A Tenuous Compromise

The compromises reached by the two sides with some mediation by Indy's Alzheimer's chapter were that CareNet would be separated on freenet so that during the evaluation period its users could not use AlzCenter or other freenet services. This change would cost the CareNet project several thousand dollars in technical assistance. In return, AlzCenter, although it would go on-line, would not be publicized as previously planned by the Alzheimer's Association chapter or the Alzheimer's Center until CareNet was over. CareNet would then give control and ownership of its IT equipment to the local chapter.

The compromise on ownership of the idea and the uniqueness of its applications, as well as the relative expenditure of effort (and therefore sharing of eventual rewards) was less cleanly settled. The center was given co-investigator status in the CareNet project, or "invited" to be so designated, depending on which side one was sitting on. Yet, years later, the CareNet side continued to emphasize its uniqueness as a health service to computer-naive users, while the AlzCenter side regarded CareNet as an "evaluation of similar (to AlzCenter) modules" that was evidence for the effectiveness of the AlzCenter design and so was justification for AlzCenter's financing and expansion. AlzCenter would remain the centerpiece of the Education and Information Transfer core of the Alzheimer's Center under federal funding.

Amicable Relations

The Alzheimer's Association chapter was in a position to mediate these conflicts because the effort would serve its own interests. Its purposes and development as an organization would be better served if both CareNet and AlzCenter could develop successfully and cooperate effectively. The chapter's main aim was to support the 8,000 families on its mailing list who were the basis of its financing.

The chapter estimated that 36,000 people had Alzheimer's in its five-county area, affecting perhaps 100,000 people. It tried to reach as many as possible with its information and guidance materials, classes, and 20 to 25 mutual support groups, which it staffed with about 550 trained lay and professional volunteers. It viewed a computer-based support system as a continuously available tool for support, especially for the caregivers who could not get to meetings of the chapter's groups. The chapter therefore not only endorsed the initial CareNet proposal, but also sat on its advisory panel, and eventually agreed to help recruit male participants, since the university center's patients were mainly women.

Implementing the Demonstration

The Alzheimer's Team

The Alzheimer's team was made up mainly of nurses, the Alzheimer's Center, and freenet. Like the already operating AIDS system, the computer programs were accessible by caregivers through home terminals that delivered information, communication, and decision support services.

The CareNet program specifically sought to improve caregivers' skill in solving the problems that commonly develop for progressively chronically ill people living at home, and to lessen their sense of isolation. It helped address issues such as whether to include the patient in social activities, where to place a person in need of residential care, and when the person's behavior indicated severe deterioration.

One hundred caregivers of Alzheimer's patients from the center clinic and the Alzheimer's Association mailing list were assigned randomly to an experimental group or to a control group for a year. The experimental group received the computer network link in their homes. The procedures and support system were similar to those in the AIDS test.

Denouement

After CareNet testing ended, there was a surge in the use of AlzCenter, presumably by former CareNet users, with over 500 interactions made within six months and a waiting list for equipment of 15 families. Some people used both the face-to-face support groups and computer program, activating each in a kind of synergy between soft and hard technology.

At that point the university Alzheimer's Center acknowledged that the main problems with its own system since inception were that only a few Alzheimer's caregivers had the equipment they needed to participate, most were not computer literate, and there was no computer support staff to train or assist them in using the system. They felt that AlzCenter had much potential but would not be well utilized. The Alzheimer's chapter would now remedy these problems. When the CareNet project was completed, the control and ownership of all the electronic equipment was turned over to the chapter as agreed.

The Alzheimer's Association, using the results of CareNet's demonstration and the national media attention it received to point out the publicity it brought to Indy, was able to win a three-year grant (endorsed by CareNet as a "technology transfer" program) from a local foundation. It would expand the AlzCenter system through more staffing, volunteer trainer training, promotion, and enough new loanable equipment for 240 users within three years.

CareNet's Users

Caregivers

An analysis of the 50 Alzheimer's caregivers who had CareNet showed they were mainly white women between the ages of 60 and 80. Half had at least a high school education and few were employed. Some had cared for a patient for as long as four years.

These users opened their computer terminal to CareNet 3,900 times during the year of the project, about 83 times each for about 13 minutes twice a week. The bulletin board was most popular, absorbing about 10 minutes each time. Of the more than 600 messages posted, the largest share were to support other group members. Other topics dealt with the situation of the Alzheimer's patient and the caregiver's own feelings about his or her circumstances. Least mentioned were caregiving skills (about 12 messages).

Private mail was also widely used, although about a third less than the bulletin board. But the most unique and technically innovative part of CareNet, the decision making module, was used least (less than 100 times, and 38 times by one individual). Most users used it only a half dozen times each during the year, taking about nine minutes each time. The information file had 500 users who were primarily interested in caring for the patient and in the disease itself. While the question-answer area was asked only 35 questions, it was read over 850 times in three-minute snippets, suggesting that the user group had many questions in common.

These caregivers said they felt more confident in making decisions about their patient, especially those who had most used both the public and private messaging modules and the question-answer service, compared with caregivers who did not have CareNet. However, the kinds of decisions they actually made were basically not different than the non-CareNet caregivers.

Cursory estimates from the study also showed that there was no difference in the health of the patients, whether or not they were transferred to nursing homes, or their remaining length of life. Nor was there a difference between the groups of caregivers in their use of formal health services. So, while there were no measurable health or health services effects from CareNet, the support it gave caregivers for smaller, in-home personal and caregiving problems may have prevented the development of larger mental or physical problems that would have been brought to health care facilities later or placed other demands on the services system.

Initially, like many professionals, caregivers too were dubious about the value of a computer. But after their experience their views changed. One man said:

> When I first heard about the computers, my first thought was "It'll never fly." I considered myself computer illiterate and felt my generation (age 73) would never be interested. Wrong! I was surprised at how easy it was to familiarize myself with it after one training session. . . . I know of no one who had a problem in learning how to use it. . . . Where else can I go to get help from so many knowledgeable and understanding caregivers through a single medium? . . . Where else can I go for the strength and encouragement to go on? . . . to say "I'm losing my coping skills, please help me?" Where else can I find out I'm not doing such a bad job as a caregiver after all?

From a woman caregiver:

> I have "talked" to my friends and fellow caregivers almost every day since getting this computer. We have made such close friends of each other and share the sorrow and the joy of what we are going through, as only we, having the same situations, would know and understand. . . . Only one thing lacking with the computer. It doesn't give *live* hugs, and we always need them.

AIDS CareNet Users

Early findings from the year-long CareNet trial for AIDS patients and their partners showed users were predominantly white young men, almost a third of whom lived alone, and about one in four of whom needed help with personal care.

The 27 computer users accessed the AIDS module about 8,400 times, 300 times on average. Typically, the link-up would last 12 or 13 minutes, occurring between 10 p.m. and 3 a.m. People first responded to their personal mail and then reviewed and responded to messages on the public bulletin board. About a fourth of the links were for either retrieving information from the encyclopedic information file or doing a decision analysis. Like the Alzheimer's caregivers, the most often used IT service was communications (more than eight of every ten uses), with the decision support module accessed in only 5 percent of uses.

These users were very individualized in their styles of seeking support. For example, they varied in their use of the information file from two minutes to over 50 hours; others used the decision support module for seven minutes to up to two hours. However, most of them did not use the kind of logical/rational approach that is implied by the compilation of accurate professional information in the information file, nor the process presented in the decision support module.

As with the Alzheimer's caregivers, the major theme running through the public message board was the sense of group feeling and mutual support. Next most common was how to manage illness symptoms, followed by existential and philosophical questions and conjectures about the future. But the AIDS users went into their private mail more often overall and for longer periods of time than into the public communication area, unlike the Alzheimer's caregivers. The enduring supportive effect of CareNet was suggested by the fact that the AIDS users went to the public forum 4,000 times, although they posted only about 750 messages, indicating that they read those messages several times.

Use of the question-answer service focused most on managing symptoms and getting services, and less on actual treatments. The relatively little time spent with the information and decision support modules was thought by the team to be because the information sections were brief and so did not require much time and the decision module might have been difficult because it provided no answers.

Individuals' Thoughts

Perhaps more significant than can be revealed by numbers is the individual experience of AIDS CareNet users. One woman said she was able to deal with more information at a pace she could control, and so she could understand it more completely. This made her more confident in taking care of herself and feeling able to confront her physician more directly than previously. Other anecdotal evidence showed how network communication seemed to encourage candor among the users. One message read. "I have been exhausted, so out of it that I couldn't even check on the system. This is no excuse because I have suffered not hearing from everyone. I miss you guys."

As AIDS users became aware of their commonalities, the experience tended to make this special disease seem more "normal," or certainly a less singular and lonely experience. When new members joined the network, it was common for users to write encouraging welcoming letters. Compared with what often happens to new individuals in face-to-face groups, these people seemed to reach out more to new members. Almost two-thirds of them eventually met face-to-face, and most kept their computers to continue using the AIDS communications and information services on freenet after the project ended.

Some of the change in participants' comfort with electronic communication is suggested in the contrast between the first and final messages on the CareNet screen. The first message arrived on the AIDS project computer when the system officially came on-line in June of 1989:

> Hi. How are you? It sure is hot outside.

The last was at the end of the evaluation in 1990:

> This good-bye stuff is making me sad. I believe that the concept of the theory of the study was to show that people who are isolated due to a disability or feel the risk involved in "coming out" about their HIV status get sicker faster. The application of this safe and anonymous (sort of) means of communication should have been a tool for learning more about what is happening to us and a way to share fears and hopes and information.
>
> I'm hoping everyone got something out of it. I did. It was a wonderful idea. And it works! I'm healthier than I would have been without it and I'm very grateful to have been one of the lucky ones chosen for the study. I think even those who didn't often contribute to the forum surely must have gained hope and knowledge from reading posts from the more outspoken ones. It's really not that much different than the world full of people, is it? Some people have an ability to express their feelings and do so. Others are quiet and most often just listen. It takes all kinds of people to make the world go 'round, and it would be pretty boring if we were all the same.
>
> Thanks to everyone for having the courage to be a part of this study.
>
> Love to all,
>
> Jonathan

The Project's Conclusions

From their preliminary reviews, the project teams concluded that the kinds of information needed by homebound people and their caregivers involved three main types: self-care and other traditional and nontraditional methods; symptom management, the meaning of symptoms, clinical markers of wellness or decline, and self-monitoring; and services, both local and national. For people living with AIDS, issues about the environment, such as uncertainty about living arrangements or composition of the household, were more critical than the presence of a caregiver. The project teams also found that the rate of physical and mental decline in a six-month period would not dramatically affect the use of a computer to support self-care for people living with AIDS.

Another conclusion was that those who monitor the system should remember that although the "active" users, those who gave and responded to messages, are a limited number, the "observing" users are more numerous. There were, in effect, dual audiences who were aware of screen conversations.

Overall, the teams felt they had showed that CareNet was feasible and was best used to support communication. It had a relatively low cost that made it particularly cost-effective—$350 per unit and approximately four hours of personnel time for installation and training.

CareNet demonstrated through its use of freenet as its parent network that existing networks could be adapted to deliver health services. Because no special programming was used, CareNet could technically be easily continued on freenet after the evaluation was over. Its advantages were that new information could be offered to and kept up-to-date for a particular user group. At the same time, individuals could retain control over what they accepted, when they used it and how often, and the extent of privacy and anonymity they desired.

Provider Issues

There were issues resulting from this new medium that the provider of expert information would have to address. Information must be offered clearly to minimize misinterpretation, and must be placed where the intended audience would access it. An effort also should be made to indicate in words or symbols something of the tone of the message, since the medium is so devoid of customary face-to-face nuance. Yet, the habit of users to return to their screens to reread the public forum speaks to what it must be conveying to them in quite personal ways.

CareNet's evaluators also concluded that health services—information, counseling, and professional advice—could be effectively delivered through this medium. But first, the real need for these services by specific potential users should be carefully evaluated, along with the capacity of the health care delivery system to supply the services, which are currently unreimbursable. Organizational issues that would have to be addressed include establishing charges, billing, liability, clinical responsibility, and the extent of integration between the community electronic network and the health facility's information and record-keeping systems.

Organization Spin-Offs

A "Virtual Organization"

As some of CareNet's users continued their electronic relationships through transfer to the Alzheimer's Association chapter, some became acquainted with the association's members. Within a few months about ten began to refer to themselves as the "computer family." Soon these men and women caregivers, ranging between 45 and 74 years old, met for lunch and continued to meet monthly. This unanticipated spin-off of CareNet suggests new possibilities of networks even among very burdened, non-"techie" people. The development of electronic groups, virtual on-line organizations, can lead to the formation of informal groups, and eventually perhaps formal organizations.

Organization Learning

After CareNet, the views of organizational leaders changed. They suggested, for example, that students in the college of nursing needed a broader understanding of computers in health services, that nursing interventions need no longer be face-to-face encounters with clients, and that decision-making support based on a rational model is not necessarily what caregivers or patients want when they manage chronic illness at home. In effect, the findings from CareNet were a window into viewpoints that are common within households. This new perspective augured changes in educational and service program development, at least in the long run.

The services of the local Alzheimer's chapter were changed too, and not only through the development of computer support services. The social workers had initially wondered whether "a computer could replace a hug," *that* was what the face-to-face support groups were all about. After CareNet, they became converted to it as a legitimate, usable substitute or supplemental service.

The staff physicians who actually used CareNet also became convinced of its community usefulness, although they were not yet in decision-making positions in their organizations to bring about program changes.

Technology Transfer and Organization Development

The issue of what to do with the two CareNet projects after the evaluations was not dealt with at the outset other than that the software was to be offered to freenet. In the case of the AIDS project, no one was willing to maintain the system. The result was ad hoc and futile efforts to keep it available to users by setting up a terminal in the gays' Homeplace and training the staff, and by allowing a graduate student nurse respond to the question-answer module at the college. These arrangements, without being an institutionalized program commitment, ended when the individuals who were immediately involved left.

The aftermath of the Alzheimer's CareNet project was constructively forced into a more organized transfer by the agreement to give the equipment and software to the Alzheimer's Association. Because CareNet's results were persuasive to the association, and it saw the possibility of strengthening member and donor support by expanding this service, it made a successful effort to get local foundation funds to institutionalize its own variation of CareNet in the AlzCenter system in conjunction with the university's Alzheimer's Center.

Without the local chapter's success at getting grant money, it is doubtful whether the AlzCenter electronic program would have been sustainable over the longer term. Its status in the interval between the end of CareNet and the startup of the Alzheimer's chapter's new grant program was tentative at best. Apart from the modules being operated by the chapter's volunteers, the university Alzheimer's Center had limited professional staff time to commit to it. The encyclopedia was therefore less often updated and the question-answer module was not regularly or quickly answered. The center also had difficulty finding grant funds for staffing and for its hopes to develop a software module for professionals, as well as obtain the equipment and technical support staff to allow placement of the technology in ten agencies that dealt with Alzheimer's families (such as social service centers and nursing homes).

Organization Expansion

The college of nursing had gained public recognition for its support of CareNet through media publicity, which enhanced its reputation in the health field. Its image was also advanced in Indy, on the university campus, and in the eyes of its wide net of collaborating groups and donors, as witnessed in its self-portrayal as a leading-edge institution. CareNet then became a way to "bootstrap" further expansion by seeking foundation and other external funds for new variations of the program.

The college as a whole, according to its five-year strategic plan, was to develop a Center for Caregiving in line with its commitment to reach out into the community. Startup funds were expected to come from a local corporation with interests in homecare equipment. This center would also house a Center for Caregiver Technology, which would now include home-based information technology.

As the successful demonstrations of CareNet came to an end, the question was, what next? How do you *extend* an innovation that seems to at least partly solve a new and growing problem, that of support for family caregivers of homebound, dependent people? To academics, who almost always end their research reports with a discussion of the limitations of the study and the need for further research, the answer was to seek more research funds for some variation of the research question.

In this case, the strategy for continuation was two-fold: to further evaluate the CareNet data, and to extend CareNet to another age group (chronically ill children) in another social group (low-income, mainly African American residents). Grant writing and grant seeking then began anew. The further issue of whether and how this potential facet of electronic home health services should or could be put into practice, which was a question of health policy, was pushed onto some future horizon.

Summary: Setting, Problems, and Strategies

Indy was wired with a freenet as a partial answer for its own efforts to bind the community in precarious fiscal and social times. This also made it hospitable to new uses for community IT. Agencies were gaining experience with information technology and the leading university accepted responsibility for its own and the community's IT development. The college of nursing recognized the outward direction of health care delivery to underserved groups and community sites and the reality that health professionals who were out in front of the new trajectory would play a role in shaping a renewed delivery system. Accordingly, it geared itself to test new ideas and to support the "fame-seeking," IT-innovating faculty it recruited. It even reinterpreted its nursing mission in terms of the "information society."

The college's institutional interests in expansion, status, and influence led it to establish relations with new community constituencies, traditional health and social service agencies, the university, new business supporters, and national foundations and research funders. All this created an enabling, fertile—but not determining or prescriptive—climate for innovation.

The idea of an electronic support system for home caregivers was fleshed out by newly recruited faculty during the process of deliberately forming network of supportive contacts, individuals who had an interpersonal expertise and interest in expanding the uses of community IT. Yet it was the college that took the initiative to seek funds and organize the design and implementation structures to bring the idea to fruition. In a broad sense, the idea became reality as a result of the confluence of problems and interests of critical stakeholders: the health care delivery system (costs, access, long-term illness, and disability), the college (institutional expansion), and nursing as a profession.

Resources

Financing the idea became successful due to new sources of demonstration and research grants from private and public sources, and as a result of reworking the IT concept into programs that met the priorities of specific funders. The necessary faculty expertise was engaged by offering career incentives, such as experience in grant development, association with known researchers, and publications. For the NIH's Nursing Research Center, for example, using IT for supporting home caregiving brought the nursing profession into the information age, and would also anchor its traditional role of providing in-home services.

Design

As an electronic network, CareNet for each project provided a database of encyclopedic information on either Alzheimer's Disease or AIDS, a decision support module, and communications services for public and private messaging. The software designs were based on feedback from the prospective users.

Sensitive design and user-friendliness for the target populations whom CareNet sought to reach—people living with AIDS and Alzheimer's caregivers—were essential, and required staff, time, training, and funds. But the precondition for success was to obtain the cooperation of the organizations that controlled access to clients, technology, and services, and the potential for continuing CareNet programs after the test periods.

Processes

Establishing workable organizational linkages required maneuvering among the shoals of collaboration and competition, cost and gain, short- and long-term relations. It meant ensuring no decline in the normal control over clients by their doctors, nurses, or social workers; no loss of resources by clinics or the university or community groups, showing how CareNet could enhance the goals of each to reach out to the community; being on the leading edge of technology and acquiring expertise in new forms of IT; and supporting a socially valued program and improving one's public image.

Some organizational qualms were neutralized by early consultations and the establishment of a wide communication network, which was renewed at frequent intervals by face-to-face meetings where CareNet's progress and problems were reported. But other enticements also smoothed and sustained cooperative relations, including money payments, IT equipment, favorable publicity, expanded clienteles, coauthorship on publications, and the hope of improved future grant-getting prospects as a result of association with CareNet.

CareNet became sustainable after its testing phase, when technology transfer was planned and when there was a preexisting organizational web with sufficient fiscal incentive and self-interest to adopt it as an ongoing program. It was thus able to continue for Alzheimer's caregivers through the local Alzheimer's Association chapter, but not for people with AIDS, who had little supportive organizational infrastructure.

Competition and partly incompatible goals did not necessarily preclude collaboration when mutual dependence for essential resources existed, as between CareNet and the university's Alzheimer's Center, which controlled access to patients. But maintaining workable ties required constant attention. Compromise over operational control was easier to reach than over invention of the concept.

Collaboration was clearly easier, longer lasting, and more beneficial to each party when organizational interests coincided, as between CareNet and the local Alzheimer's Association chapter. The chapter's reward was good publicity, improved grant-getting, and program expansion. The college had ready access to caregivers and saw CareNet evolve into an ongoing and enlarged program.

The college of nursing, as a result of CareNet, improved its grant-getting prospects for research and program funds and gained from publicity showing it as a high-tech, yet community-oriented institution, an image that appealed to many business and other donors.

Results

Unexpected findings from the CareNet trials revealed that the most used and useful electronic services were the communication tools, which fostered a group sense and created a "virtual community" among users. The more rational tool, the decision support module, was used least.

The experience of the Alzheimer's Association chapter seemed to show that caregivers used both face-to-face meetings and on-line communication to seek mutual support; one did not preclude the other, and in fact, CareNet fostered the development of the "computer family" lunch group. CareNet also showed that although "active" users were limited in number, there were many more "observing" users who also seemed to benefit from the on-line information and sense of community of the active users.

The development and at least short-term success of CareNet was mothered by ready access to a variety of resources and supporting structures. Even so, it was a long and difficult experience that required continued organized attention to be sustained. When the richness of supports is sparse, the effort to develop community IT is far more arduous and time-consuming, and the outcome is less secure, as the next cases show.

References

American Public Health Association. 1992. *Public Health Report Card*. Washington, DC: APHA.

Bureau of the Census. 1988. *County and City Data Book*. Washington, DC: Department of Commerce.

National Public Telecomputing Network. 1993. *The Bluebook*. Cleveland, OH: NPTN.

Office of Technology Assessment (OTA). 1984. *Technology and Aging in America*. Washington, DC: U.S. Congress.

———. 1990. *Confused Minds, Burdened Families*. Washington, DC: U.S. Congress.

Weinberger, M., et al. 1993. "Expenditures in Caring for Patients with Dementia Who Live at Home." *American Journal of Public Health 83*(3): 338–40.

SECTION B

Social Support for Outcasts and Neighborhoods

Is there a person among you who will offer someone a stone when they ask for bread, or a snake when they ask for fish? . . . Always treat others as you would like them to treat you.

Words of Jesus, quoted in Matthew
The New English Bible,

CHAPTER

7

REACHING OUT WITH INFORMATION TECHNOLOGY

Educating Children, Engaging Elders

INFORMATION TECHNOLOGY is spreading across the land, inevitably affecting, if not connecting, every age group and every aspect of social life. The large-scale players and most advantaged groups are reaping most of its benefits (OTA 1993). In some places, efforts are being made in social and government sectors to extend the benefits of IT to local communities and to less advantaged people. The first efforts to reach out though IT have meant, as in the health field, IT support for professional providers of services, emphasizing information transfer, not the exploration of communication and organizational possibilities on behalf of or by community groups. Nonetheless, in addition to technology innovations, social creations—social or soft technology—are emerging.

Linking the Age Scale

Information technology is becoming a part of everyday activity at both ends of the age scale, but not at an even pace or in an equitable fashion. Children and elders are using computers, sometimes combined with telecommunications, to do required tasks like education and self-support and to engage in free-time essentials like entertainment, communication, and hobbies. Occasionally, the two groups find common cause in using IT together, as the next vignette (Chapter 8) illustrates.

Early Education

Computers have been in American classrooms for over 30 years. In the early 1990s, there was one computer for every 20 students, two to three times more than in the mid-eighties. The use of information-laden compact discs (CD-ROMs), which now house encyclopedias, books, and videodiscs (like one on the San Francisco earthquake), are multiplying in the nation's 15,000 school districts. Outside links through satellite dishes and computer wirelines tripled in the early nineties, and are likely to mushroom before the end of the century as the information infrastructure develops with new legislation to support connections to schools across the country. The leaders in this quickened technology pace, not surprisingly, were the affluent suburbs (Strothman 1991; OTA 1985).

Information Banks and Competition vs. Discovery and Collaboration

Even with this overall technological capacity, computer-based pedagogy of the early nineties continued to emphasize the transmission of knowledge and information, contrary to the way children learn outside the classroom, where they grasp new ideas and ways of doing things through the verbal and contextual support of adults and peers (DeVillar and Faltis 1991). Learning occurs when students actively build on their own knowledge and cooperatively interact with others. This student-centered and inquiry-based process is critical in designing technological approaches to education (Bell and Stern 1994).

The prevalent approach of drill and practice exercises and encouragement of individual competition make the teacher a transmitter of information and skills. This worries some educators who see an increasing reliance on prepackaged software by teachers who, under severe fiscal pressures, have little time to evaluate its real educational worth and become more like manipulators and coordinators of tools rather than creators and judges of educational processes (Apple 1993).

In the world of the professions, commerce, and government, some leaders recognize that the acceleration of information growth makes attempts to simply transmit knowledge obsolete. The skills to support constant, life-long learning are essential to build sustainable quality in the lives of individuals, including the ability to learn and act in concert with others in complex and changing circumstances. The world will never grow simpler nor more predictable. Rather than use IT as repositories of knowledge, we could use the technologies to support communication and provide discovery-oriented learning opportunities for students working together in small groups, with an adult or more capable peer (DeVillar and Faltis 1991).

This approach, which encourages collaboration, critical inquiry, and problem solving, is more relevant to real-life learning and to the diverse, interdependent world to which children and adults must constantly adjust and contribute. It would be best to prepare them to use IT as a new tool to help them address social and economic problems, and related health problems in their communities.

IT Equity

Instructional habits will need to move beyond current teacher-centered delivery systems that use computers as knowledge-dispensing machines—like the conventional emphasis on information in the health care system—to begin to develop IT's potential for childhood education (McCluskey 1994). More will be needed than placing equal numbers of computers in schools. To ensure IT equity among school districts, schools, ethnic groups, and genders, the IT capacity of poorer schools needs special support. Soft technology—people, knowledge, and organizations—will have to balance the hard technology. This includes better software, more qualified teachers and computer-related texts, funds for machine repair, technical support, and retraining. Congressional legislation to promote IT equity was introduced in the early nineties, but had limited chance for adequate funding because of stringent budget limits (Bingaman 1993). Without technological equity, the academic achievement gap between groups can only widen, and that gap will threaten the prospects for employment, community inclusiveness, and ultimately, health in the future.

Seniors Learning

At the other end of the age scale, computers are making life more comfortable for growing numbers of elders, extending their senses and supporting ordinary activities when their biological limits are restrictive in the later decades of life. For example, voice-output capabilities on calculators, thermometers, and scales can help the poor-sighted, and interactive computers allow at-home shopping, banking, bill paying, and control of home safety and security devices for those with limited mobility (Ogozolek 1992).

Although IT can provide these kinds of self-support tools for everyday living, there are at least two reasons why they will not be extensively used in the foreseeable future. One is that IT equity cannot exist among elders as long as poverty remains significant among certain groups of them. Over one in five Hispanic elders is poor; a third of native American and African American elders are poor; and women of all races are disproportionately represented among the poor (Dychtwald and Flower 1989). A second reason that in-home support with IT may be limited in its use is that most elders do not need or want to be homebound; they want to continue to go out and have contact with the world (Tingay 1988).

Whether frail or robust, the elderly are able to learn to use computers to extend their contacts, and they are willing to take on some of the tasks that once meant dependence on professionals and others (Eilers

1989; Edwards and Englehardt 1989; Weisman 1983; OTA 1985). For example, a study of over 100 better-educated elderly people showed they felt able and willing to use a computer as a substitute and supplement for personal communications with their pharmacist or doctor. As one woman said, "I feel the computer can give you much information that you don't always get from a physician. They usually feel that you won't understand what they're saying." Elders, who make up about 12 percent of Americans, get over a third of the 1.5 billion prescriptions written each year (Ogozolek 1992).

An Elders' Network

If IT can make home living more convenient for elders, it can also take them out of the bounds of the house, literally and electronically, when they choose. SeniorNet, a computer network for elders, was begun as an experiment in the mid-eighties by a nonprofit organization. By the early nineties it had several dozen sites across the country at which elders could learn about and use computers for a small membership fee. Elders could also access the network for a monthly fee of about $10 (SeniorNet 1991).

An Advantaged Group

SeniorNet's more than 4,000 members were mainly between 65 and 70 years old, and two-thirds owned computers. The typical member was a man with some college education and a yearly income of $20–$30,000. He was married and living in a suburban single family home (Schwarz and Schwarz 1991). By contrast, the typical member who used the SeniorNet computer sites was an urban woman with an income between $10,000 and $20,000, and not likely to own a computer. She was also more socially outgoing than her suburban male counterpart.

Net Effects

In general, SeniorNet members used computers for writing and personal finances. But they joined the electronic network (in addition to using the computer sites) for social reasons: to learn and keep their minds active, to meet other people in person and on-line, and to "keep up with" their children and grandchildren.

These interests were evident in the favored services offered on-line. The overwhelming uses were not for information access, but for the discussion forums and electronic mail. IT in the hands of these elders had further local social spin-offs. The members helped others, both adults and children, learn to use computers. They donated computer time and services to community groups or individuals, writing club reports, providing computer support for several nonprofit organizations such as food aid groups, libraries, and churches, and helping medically indigent people obtain services and disabled and elderly persons do personal accounting (Schwarz and Schwarz 1991).

Connecting with Community Life

Getting the right kinds of help to individuals at the right time is an especially complicated problem in the United States, with its myriad, often overlapping and fragmented, and not necessarily adequate spectrum of available services and resources. Only a limited share of people who are eligible for services actually receive them (GAO 1992). Some of this ineffectiveness is the result of underfunding of programs; but there are other reasons as well, including a person's not knowing about a useful program or how to apply for it. To the extent that deficient information is a barrier, IT can bring light and guidance through the thicket of social and community services.

Helping Individuals

Provider Support

In the 1980s, most uses of IT supported service *providers* and did so to give service to *individuals* as consumers of information, not to community organizations for purposes beyond information. For example, counselors were guided by computer programs in talk therapies for clients with mental health, work stress, or alcohol problems (Smith 1987; Meier and Sampson 1989; Arbona and Perrone 1989; Blazyk et al. 1987).

Another variation was information and referral services, such as one operated to provide services to older people in a Georgia county. There, personnel had computerized, updated listings of 1,500 services for the aged that could be searched when help was requested by elderly people. As with similar systems, this one failed because of both hardware problems and "soft"—organizational—problems such as lack of computer consultants, staff attrition, and new staff not having the training to use the computerized system. In other words, there was not enough back-up support for the providers; the soft technology, the social infrastructure, was not as developed as the hard technology (GAO 1991).

Consumer Access

A step beyond having providers give information to consumers were the new electronic systems to allow consumers to find what they wanted for themselves—an automated computer network for disabled people with files for self-help resources, for example (Madara et al. 1988). In the nineties, emerging technologies, such as touchscreens and compact discs (CD-ROMs) made possible another form of direct electronic access to community information resources: interactive kiosks. In an agricultural community with many Southeast Asian refugees in California, the county's department of social services created an interactive touchscreen system to guide county citizens through the process of applying for Medicaid and Aid to Families with Dependent Children programs. Developed with help from a private firm, the hardware and development costs were $3.2 million, but were expected to save over $100 million by the end of the century by reducing errors and improving efficiency (Strothman 1991).

Beyond Information

Churches and libraries are historical constants in almost every American community. People claim church or synagogue membership at about the same high level as at mid-century—almost 60 percent (OTA 1990). Americans continue to give more money and time to religious groups than to all other voluntary organizations put together (Bellah et al. 1985).

But in an extended period of budget austerity, churches, libraries, and other community organizations have had to prove their worth anew to their constituencies, to extend their reach, and to find new ways to support themselves. Accordingly, churches have become involved in collaborating with other local service groups, and libraries have expanded their services. Information technology provides one important set of strategic tools for the task (National Heart, Lung, and Blood Institute 1992).

The public library system in Maryland planned to electronically unify its 21 local systems and link them all into the national and international Internet, the "network of networks," before the end of the century. Every citizen would be able, through the local library or home computer or television set, to access books and request loans. They would be able to read articles and have them delivered, obtain service agency and government information, including health information, legislation, and job listings, and communicate with others for queries and discussions. Based on a Maryland state survey, the people most needing easy access to self-support information, are older people, women, those with less than a high school education, and people with limited incomes. These are all potential new users of expanded library services. Alongside the widening of the network, funds were provided for staff training and public education to enable effective use of the system (State Library 1992).

Organization

Moving beyond information access, an old neighborhood church in a people-dense, deprived area of San Francisco reached into the life of its community by adding new IT tools to do its work. Enriching its support and survival services to its local immigrant and homeless clientele, the church opened a computer learning center in the late eighties, with the help of technology entrepreneurs (Bunnell 1988). The center offered IT programs for all age groups, ranging from basic computer literacy to job skills training to digital music and computer art. Many dozens of volunteers were also trained to support the 1,000 students who attended courses in the first year. About four out of ten adults, all earning less than $12,000 a year, completed their coursework (Computers and You 1991).

A further variation on the idea of community-based information technology, the Community Interest Computer Consultancy (CICC), was developed in the late eighties in Melbourne, Australia. With seed money from local foundations, its purpose was to help community organizations make decisions about and effectively use information technology, as well as to promote public debate on the social impacts of IT (CICC 1985).

The CICC was an advisory service and clearinghouse on community IT issues and activities, its program based initially on a local survey. It produced educational manuals and held training workshops and seminars. Through government funds, the CICC provided job training for young people and supported the development of other community services—for example, by guiding the computerization of the state's 21 community legal centers, helping set up a women's health information center that required IT capability, and assisting the development of a public interest group, the Telecommunications Policy Action Group (*Critical Edge* 1987; Community Technology 1988).

The CICC thus extended community information technology beyond access to information and communication between individuals, to support for community development, and helped organizations that would provide local services and advocate public interest policies. Unfortunately, its mission was cut short by the stringencies of government budget cuts and the limited funds of its community-based, nonprofit organizational clientele.

The vignettes in the next two chapters reveal laborious but successful efforts in two U.S. communities to link age groups and reach out to support those who are cast out of the mainstream of community life.

References

Apple, M. 1993. *Official Knowledge*. London: Routledge.

Arbona, C., and P. Perrone. 1989. "Use of the Computer in Counseling College Students." *Computers in Human Services* 5 (3–4): 99–112.

Bell, P., and J. Stern. 1994. "NII in Education: Access Isn't Enough." *CPSR Newsletter* 12 (2): 4–6.

Bellah, R., et al. 1985. *Habits of the Heart*. New York: Harper and Row.

Bingaman, L. 1993. *The Technology and Education Act of 1993.* (S. 1040). Washington, DC: U.S. Congress.

Blazyk, S., et al. 1987. "Computer-Based Case Management for the Elderly." *Computers in Human Services* 2 (1–2): 63–77.

Bunnell, D. 1988. "Taking IT to the Streets." *PC World*, August.

Community Interest Computer Consultancy (CICC). 1985. Management Committee. *Proposal for a Community Interest Computer Consultancy*. Melbourne, Victoria, Australia: Royal Melbourne Institute of Technology and Victorian Council of Social Service, April.

Community Technology. 1988. *Social Justice and Information Technology*. Report to the Stegley Foundation. Melbourne, Victoria, Australia, May.

Computers and You. 1991. *Computers and You: A Fact Sheet*. San Francisco: Computers and You.

Critical Edge. 1987. 1: 2–4.

DeVillar, R., and C. Faltis. 1991. *Computers and Cultural Diversity: Restructuring for School Success*. Albany, NY: State University of New York Press.

Dychtwald, K., and J. Flower. 1989. *Age Wave: The Challenges and Opportunities of an Aging America*. Los Angeles, CA: Jeremy P. Tarcher.

Edwards, R., and K. Englehardt. 1989. "Microprocessor-Based Innovations and Older Americans: AARP Survey Results and Their Implications for Service Robotics." *International Journal of Technology and Aging* 2 (1): 43–55.

Eilers, M. 1989. "Older Adults and Computer Education: Not to Have a Closed Door." *International Journal of Technology and Aging* 2 (1): 57–76.

General Accounting Office (GAO). 1991. *Outreach Services in Federal Programs*. Washington, DC: U.S. Congress.

———. 1992. *Early Intervention*. Washington, DC: U.S. Congress, 7 April.

Madara, E., et al. 1988. "The Computerized Self-Help Clearinghouse: Using High Tech to Promote High Touch Support Networks." *Computers in Human Services* 3 (4): 39–54.

McCluskey, L. 1994. "Technology and Education." *Phi Delta Kappan* 75 (7): 550–52.

Meier, S., and J. Sampson. 1989. "Use of CAI in the Prevention of Alcohol Abuse." *Journal of Drug Education* 19 (3): 245–56.

National Heart, Lung, and Blood Institute. 1992. "Church and Community-Based Stroke Prevention Programs." Special Edition. *Infomemo*, 4–10.

Office of Technology Assessment (OTA). 1985. *Technology and Aging in America*. Washington, DC: U.S. Congress.

———. 1993. *Making Government Work: Delivery of Government Services.* Washington, DC: U.S. Congress.

Ogozolek, V. 1992. The "Automated Pharmacist." Dissertation. Worcester State College, Worcester, MA.

Schwarz, W., and M. Schwarz. 1992. *Summary of SeniorNet Baseline Survey 1988–1990*. SeniorNet Research Report #2a. San Francisco: SeniorNet, April.

SeniorNet. 1991. *SeniorNet Fact Sheet.* San Francisco: SeniorNet, June.

Smith, J. 1987. "The Effectiveness of a Computerized Self-Help Stress Coping Program with Adult Males." *Computers in Human Services* 1 (1–2): 37–49.

State Library and Information Services. 1992. *The Seymour Plan.* Baltimore, MD: SLIS.

Strothman, J. E. 1991. *Interactive Multimedia: Promise and Pitfalls.* Paper presented at the COMDEX O.P.E.N. Conference, Bethesda Marriott Hotel, Bethesda, MD, fall.

Tingay, M. 1988. *Attitudes and Technologies—Striving to Match New Electronic Information Products and Services to the Needs and Interests of Elderly People.* Aspen Forum Report #7. New York: Aspen Institute.

Weisman, S. 1983. "Computer Games for the Frail Elderly." *The Gerontologist* 23 (4): 361–63.

CHAPTER

8

AN ELECTRONIC SAFETY NET IN SOUTHCITY

Wired Churches and Mobile Teams to Meet Street People

EVEN IN a bright southern sun, the small office up a steep staircase behind Union Baptist Church looked as poor as the community it served on the south side of Southcity. It seemed hardly the place to nurture a vision of information technology. These wired tools were becoming crucial for salvaging the people and communities spread across the poor, urban region of this mainly affluent metropolitan area of two and a half million people. The Clearinghouse for Emergency Aid to the Community (CHEC) was "an electronic tool to help organize the helpers . . . so that we can empower the poor, needy, and homeless to become self-sufficient, thereby creating a more just society. . . . After all, we are all dealing with the most precious thing in the world: life." These were the words of Christian Help Center of metropolitan Southcity head, Sister Marie.

Sister Marie wanted to help the center's church and human services collaborators understand and adopt new IT tools that could support them in attending to the growing day-to-day needs of the homeless and poor. At first glance, IT seemed a complex and superfluous luxury. Yet, as Sister Marie put it, "Right now, we're taking from people their dignity, time, and energy, making them go from place to place to ask for help, the left hand not knowing what the right hand is doing. We need to give to them the means for a way out, an effective, coordinated way."

The City and Its People

At least a quarter of Southcity's half-million people were poor, living in neighborhoods with deteriorating housing and high rates of crime, drugs, and infant mortality. By the early nineties, after a decade of economic boom, the jobs and housing available to the poor had declined. Development leveled neighborhoods without replacing what was lost, even though the city owned 23 public housing sites. In the early eighties, when Sister Marie arrived from Kansas City where she had worked with the homeless, about 3,300 people sought shelter each night. Ten years later, 15,000 asked for a bed. The number was growing by 20 percent a year, as Southcity became one of the least-housed cities in the country.

Projected economic growth would intensify these circumstances, a local task force for the homeless reported. Two-thirds of the homeless were African American, another tenth Hispanic. Most were men, but in the nineties, there was a rapid increase in the number of homeless pregnant women and single women with children. HIV rates were high, especially among black men. The statewas not highly supportive of the city's people. It put the population among the more disadvantaged in the nation with low levels of investment in education, medical insurance, prenatal care, and public assistance. The school graduation rate was almost the lowest in the country, and violent crime and child poverty were among the highest (APHA1992; Bureau of the Census 1988).

Homelessness and Health

Homeless people, subject to even more problems of daily living and vulnerability to disease than other disadvantaged people face, have the added burdens of having no place to rest when ill, no place to store their belongings, including medications, and no certainty of obtaining a sound diet. They are exposed not only to inclement weather but also to crowded shelters among possibly infectious and abusive or even violent people. The roots of homelessness—job loss, abusive partners, substance abuse, financial loss from divorce or medical problems—further complicate their lives and expose them to seek escape through drugs and alcohol, and result in consequent problems, including HIV infection. Their present plight, if not their past, often makes them feel alienated and distrustful even of those who would merit their trust.

The Christian Help Center and Its Partners

The Christian Help Center was organized in the mid-1980s under the local Council of Churches to obtain public funds to meet the emergency needs of people who lived on the street and literally were knocking on church doors for food and shelter. Having done "street organizing" in the sixties, Sister Marie brought the downtown religious groups and churches together to coordinate their efforts in the Christian Help Center. It grew to a $200,000 operation by the early nineties.

Sister Marie also began meeting with the larger religious emergency help agencies who were having coordination problems—Central Baptist,

Mainstreet Presbyterian, Christian Aid (the protestant charity), and St. John Society (the Catholic charity). Sister Marie pointed out the efficiencies of businesses that used IT effectively. These religious organizations, which had some acquaintance with computers for in-house purposes, discussed a more sophisticated way of improving their work of trying to support the outcasts of Southcity using an electronic network.

CHEC's Beginnings

This computer network would contain lists of all available resources in the metropolitan area for emergency aid, such as housing and shelter, rent funds, food, clothing and medical care, job training, and transportation support from public and private nonprofit sources. It would be kept up-to-date and would allow each agency that was linked to it to know whether and how another agency had helped a particular individual. The system, to be known as the Clearinghouse for Emergency Aid to the Community, CHEC, would also generate a variety of reports to determine such things as overall cost of aid, unmet needs, and shelter vacancies, and would provide an account to sponsors. The "dream" was to "get all the computers and agencies talking to each other."

Development Controversies

But information technology does not talk unless people want it to do so. The initial issue was whether the sponsors should spend money and time developing CHEC rather than helping the poor. The aggressive search for funds by the center helped remedy most of that problem. A more subtle and recurring issue, even for religious and help-giving groups, was who would get credit if CHEC were a success. None of the groups wanted necessarily to await the biblical promise, "Great is your reward in heaven," since getting credit for success would improve money-raising prospects in the here-and-now.

Once they had agreed to move forward, another issue was the design of a common application form for aid seekers. What minimum information should be required? For example, was marital status a necessary item? The moral overtones and religious importance of this issue differed among the groups, depending on whether they believed that single mothers "deserved" help. They finally agreed not to ask the question. Furthermore, subjective judgments about the appearance, attitude, or behavior of clients were not allowed in the record—only basic, verifiable information.

Other issues were not resolvable, such as the input of individual client information into the system. The Christian Aid charity decided that it could not morally share its clients' files, even with the signed consent form that CHEC clients would use when they asked for aid. As a result, the charity dropped out of the core sponsor group, with some suspicion by the others that retaining client names had to do with "territoriality." Individual clients were the justification for the organization's existence and continued funding. Christian Aid went on to develop its own network modeled after CHEC.

Later in the 1980s, as CHEC became operational, more serious disagreements arose. Should such resources as birth control and abortion services be listed in the on-line database? Should the local AIDS support group, including gay organizations, be part of the system? Central Baptist was adamant about excluding these resources. It was joined by other fundamentalist and Catholic members of the citywide Council of Churches that housed the center. Each cited religious positions for taking an absolute stance on these issues. "We use theology a lot to justify what we don't want to do," were the words of Sister Marie, who disagreed with her colleagues.

The result of this zero-sum conflict was that by the early 1990s, the Church Help Center, with its CHEC network members, split off from the Council of Churches and became an independent entity. The remaining CHEC members, including some fundamentalist and Catholic groups, resolved the controversial reproductive and sex-related issues by agreeing to not impose their own values on everyone who was in need of the resources they controlled.

Resource Problems

The moral and ethical issues were settled, but the organizational problems had only begun. The center's assumption was that the entire CHEC system, hardware and software, would move with it. This was not so. They had to start from square one. One result was the austere office behind Union Baptist. The center no longer had the core administrative support of the Council of Churches.

To sustain itself financially, the center "played every game in the book." By presenting its services program and the purposes of CHEC, and by documenting the unmet needs of Southcity's poor and homeless people with CHEC's information base and reporting tools, it retained almost all of its network subscribers and got commitments of budget support from a variety of new sources. The center's $300,000 annual budget in the early nineties was met in 5 percent chunks from each of three sources: individual donations, endowment funds, and small community grants. Another 20 percent came from federal sources for emergency housing and energy assistance, and a community development block grant. Two-thirds of the budget came from the United Way.

Half the Church Help Center budget paid for administration, including Sister Marie, who doubled as head and caseworker, another case worker, a secretary and intake coordinator, and the CHEC system manager. The other $150,000 went directly to clients seeking aid. This primarily paid for emergency housing expenses, and was contingent on individuals who were physically able to attend four financial management classes. Clients did so in large groups of 70 to 100, and most went to all four sessions.

In the early nineties, the center and its collaborating network paid out over a half-million dollars in aid to help about 38,000 people. But they had to turn away another 4,800 who needed about $1.5 million.

The CHEC System

In addition to the cost of the manager's salary, CHEC cost about $1,250 a year to maintain and earned $5,000 in fees. However, when the center restarted independently, funds were not the only problem. Another major issue was technical support. For the first nine months as a freestanding program, the essential reprogramming and development of CHEC—minus about six years of archival files retained by the Council of Churches—was done by a lay preacher. After his disappearance, he was found out to be more interested in reselling the CHEC package than in customizing it to carry out charitable work—a better entrepreneur than a good neighbor. He left no documentation on the system he had set up, leaving his successor to learn its structure by trial and error.

Fortunately, his replacement was a newly retired federal government "hacker" who wanted to use his skills for the good of the community and who became personally committed to revamping CHEC. He wanted to turn it into a system that was capable of not only getting computers talking to each other, but also allowing users to define a single responsible agency for each client (a primary coordinator) if they collectively so decided, and to talk to each other, as well as to the center, by electronic mail.

CHEC's growth proceeded with deliberate slowness, involving its user organizations face-to-face. As CHEC's IT specialist soon learned, "It's only going to work if everybody plays. . . . The problem is to slowly convince them that it's worth their time." Within six months the center had a new manual to document its reorganized system and train its users, while further changes and improvements evolved.

CHEC's explicit aim was to provide church outreach ministries and human services agencies with the means to collect and share information and referral services. Its database inventoried almost 450 service agencies in metropolitan Southcity and updated them on a monthly basis. This was done in a rather paradoxical, "low-tech" fashion, often by calling many dozens of agencies to ask whether their services had changed. This costly process was necessary because CHEC did not have the technological capability to accomplish the task electronically. More importantly, the 450 agencies were not subscribers to CHEC services.

Operating Issues

The CHEC system had two subscriber categories to accommodate the degree of interest and resources of its organizational constituents. The ONLINE option, at $200 a year, provided all available services: community resources availability information, such as health services and housing vacancies; technical assistance; reports on resources, applicants, and transactions, including unmet needs; and an electronic mail service with the Church Help Center. The resources in the 450-agency database, for example, could be listed by name, area served, county, funding source, or type of need, and reports could be made of systemwide financial or services transactions in a variety of formats. About a dozen agencies chose the on-line option; start-up capacity costs were the limiting factors.

An equal number chose a second, the ON-SITE option. At $125 yearly, the center provided a diskette of updated resource availability listings that was mailed to subscribers each month. All members received on-site installation and training as well as support services by telephone.

There were a number of reasons why the electronic network was so small in contrast to its potential organizational users and apparent need for coordinating a vast array of services to a clientele with many unmet needs. The main reason, at least for the small churches, was economic, flavored with computer phobia. The necessary hardware was a fairly fast and sophisticated 386 microprocessor computer and modem connected to a telephone line, which often meant installing a second line at some sites and new wiring in others. The ON-SITE users needed the same equipment minus the modem. These investments in infrastructure cost more than many small agencies could afford.

To help bring the smaller churches and agencies into the support network, the center attempted, with modest success, to get large local companies like the gas utility to donate their old personal computers. It also hoped to get a major modem producer to donate modems to all current and prospective members. In such negotiations, however, the center was in a double bind. To justify such requests, it had to show that it had an organizational clientele sufficiently large to attract at least the public relations if not commercial interests of profit makers. But it could not expand its network to create that clientele very easily as long as the technology was beyond the capacity of low-budget, nonprofit agencies.

Other intergroup issues continued to interrupt the creation of a unified network. For example, initially the local homeless task force was an avid user of CHEC. But once it secured a base of funding, it developed its own electronic net, modeled after CHEC.

Sharing files on individuals, such that one agency could learn about the needs and services provided to specific people, continued to be a problem due to agencies wanting to retain control of their "own" clients. Yet, most agencies wanted to be able to track clients in this way, and maintained that they were in business to meet people's needs in the fullest way possible. They also wanted customized monthly reports from the center on their own services, clients, and payouts, as well as similar data for the network as a whole, some of which required a sharing of records. The related question of retaining confidentiality in a wide network remained a concern for the center, although it believed that with goodwill and time-consuming effort, the technical means to achieve it was possible.

Another continuing problem in maintaining unity was the turnover of personnel in the member agencies. Not only did this require repeated training at agency sites, it could also mean that, depending on the computer attitudes or stereotypes of new staff, the entire link might be dropped. To avoid such breaks, the center had to maintain constant communication with its client groups, frequent "hand holding," training, and re-education.

A Contingent Future

Many of the issues involved in expanding and strengthening CHEC could be addressed with a larger base budget to hire staff to negotiate, train, and promote the network, and to upgrade the center's technology with a faster and larger system. The needed technology was estimated at $25,000 in the early nineties. This could move the center toward its vision of linking all public and private human services agencies serving disadvantaged people in each of metropolitan Southcity's 11 counties, as one county had already done using CHEC's software. The hope was for each agency to link with a central system operator and its central database containing every agency's resources, every person served, and every person with unmet needs who had asked for aid. All subscribers would also be able to communicate with the dozens or hundreds of agencies in the electronic net. Sister Marie's vision was that agencies would be "human services brokers for people without making them shop all around town." Together these agencies would make a case for the kinds of resources people needed, and with clear documentation and accountability they would persuade policymakers to support progressive changes in the region.

Whatever the reality of the dream, the center did expect to be able to enlarge its technological capacity to support a larger network, customize reports and services, and develop electronic mail among its member groups. When it had achieved its feasible limit, under the constraints of economic realities and organizational politics, it would be content to turn CHEC over to another organization or have it independently incorporated.

A Partner in Health: Mobile Services

On one of CHEC's computer screens, if the user searched for medical services in the poorest, least adequately housed areas of Southcity, she would find agency information file #398, the St. Francis Mobile Health Program, an ON-SITE subscriber. Its health care practitioners, using a fleet of four vans and a 33-foot Healthmobile, traveled to sites that became crossroads for homeless people—some 80 shelters, soup kitchens, churches, drug detoxification centers, parks, and public clinics. It brought services to clients, rather than having clients come to St. Francis Hospital for scheduled appointments. St. Francis had found in a community study, that

> It is difficult, if not impossible, to schedule diagnostic services or follow-up care because homeless people do not have money or transportation. They follow meals, job leads, and shelter vacancies rather than medical advice about controlling blood sugar, receiving prenatal care, or getting T-cell counts. A mobile population requires mobile health services, and mobile health services require a mobile information system.

The need for a mobile information system to support the organization and operation of Mobile Services, led it to develop HEALTH, a software program for laptop computers tied to a central computer at the program's office. According to the Mobile Service head, it was designed so that

> . . . it won't bite you. It walks you through the system step-by-step. [Health care providers] can be nurses and doctors, not computer experts, unless they want to be. . . . And, at the sites [where care is rendered] HEALTH and CHEC are everything you need to help a patient.

Mobile Services, Inc.

Mobile Services began in the mid-eighties when a few staff from St. Francis Hospital volunteered their evenings to help prepare meals at some of Southcity's downtown shelters for the homeless. The medical needs of the people were evident and the staff began to offer limited medical care.

After a series of organizational changes at St. Francis, Mobile Services was incorporated, making it eligible for federal funds in 1988, and relieving St. Francis, now the St. Francis Health System of Metropolitan Southcity, of some of the burden of supporting uncompensated health care.

Five years later, Mobile Services had 40 paid employees, excluding doctors, over 200 volunteers, many of whom were doctors who backed up the nurse practitioner staff, an operating budget of over $2 million, and a downtown office newly renovated by donated services from business and philanthropic groups in an area of "trashed out" buildings. It was located on a bright site, yet was protected by a tight security system.

Computers for Community Work

And it had HEALTH, its customized laptop software for patient records, client tracking, case management, and reporting. Each mobile team—usually one or two nurse practitioners, a health advocate, a laboratory worker, sometimes a social worker, and perhaps a health educator or AIDS or immunization specialist (usually nurses)—would take with them a laptop computer, portable printer, and modem, as well as other wiring to accommodate the often inadequate electrical setup at the delivery sites. About 8,000 to 9,000 people were served in over 50,000 episodes of care each year. They generally mirrored the homeless population: somewhat more men than women, although increasingly more women and children. About two-thirds were African American, and many were in the potentially most productive years of their lives (20 to 45 years old). Most came to get medical treatment for both acute and chronic conditions, while increasing numbers came for HIV testing—with a high rate of return to get the results (38 percent)—and for prenatal and young child care along with WIC (Women, Infants', and Children's Supplemental Food Program) services.

HEALTH was designed to take account of the complexities of this style of health services. At a site, the health advocate would print out a patient record on the service's own form; it showed previous contacts the person had with the service. Most of the 15,000 records in the database showed patients using the service once a year on average. The health care provider wrote the specifics of the encounter on the hard copy; the form was then taken back to the office where data entry personnel typed it into desktop computers within about 24 hours. At the site, the advocate could also call up the CHEC database and find information to help refer an individual to other resources. Using the battery power of the laptop, a caseworker could also take it outside the site when the facility was too crowded and use the CHEC system on the street, "taking health care to the curbside."

The Origin of HEALTH

HEALTH began in the late eighties as Mobile Services was undergoing a growth spurt. Its new administrator, with a background as a business and computer consultant, found herself attempting to compile patient service data for her grant reports "the old-fashioned way," by hand, even as the delivery sites began to multiply. After visiting the sites to learn what was needed to streamline operations, she reviewed numerous computer software programs, all of which seemed inadequate until she found one that was set up by another southern city's health care for the homeless program. Building on that package in collaboration with the software firm license holder, she wrote HEALTH.

By the mid-nineties, the Mobile Services laptop system would be upgraded with the necessary hardware and software to allow it to communicate with and among the mobile units, with its office and the Church Help Center office, and with its own parent organization, St. Francis Health Care Outreach, Inc.

Corporate Parents

St. Francis Outreach was one of a number of new incorporated units of the larger St. Francis Health System, following the pattern of health care restructuring that began in the 1980s. These changes evolved from the pressures of limited payments from Medicare under the new prospective payment system, from increased competition from profit-making hospitals, and from the phenomena of "creaming" (hospitals refusing treatment to noninsured patients) and "patient dumping" (sending uninsured people to public and nonprofit sites, as the numbers of poor and uninsured people grew) (Milio 1993).

The corporations of St. Francis Health Care Outreach were two nonprofit hospitals that were longtime medical providers in Southcity; St. Francis Foundation, whose task was to obtain grants and contributions for the system; and three profit-making units—St. Francis Administrative Services, Real Estate Management Services, and Clinical Services—that sold their expertise to the other corporate units. This strategic reorganization, spun off from the original hospital, came from the mother institution, the Sisters of St. Francis, founded over a century earlier to "respond to the health needs of the community and to serve the poor."

Health Care Outreach

The corporate mission given to St. Francis Health Care Outreach was to provide "care for the poor and disadvantaged and . . . form connections among persons, resources, and opportunities in order to most effectively respond to unmet needs," devising "new alternative models of care" that were low cost and replicable in the system.

Mobile Services was the first program to accomplish this mission, with its $2 million budget. Other new outreach programs were for elders, Hispanics, and Asians (with a combined budget of less than a million dollars) and were located at fixed site clinics.

The outreach organization did more than meet the widely recognized humanitarian needs of Southcity's disadvantaged people. It was—as were its sister corporations—a form of "unbundling" services from their previous hospital base—for which compensation from third party payers was low or nonexistent—to an entity that was eligible for a variety of public funds, and was visible enough to encourage large corporate and other private contributions. And, it was a contemporary way to carry out the century-old mission of the religious Sisters.

The volunteer forerunner of Mobile Services had been transformed in the later eighties, under a decision of the St. Francis Health System, into an incorporated community coalition for specific purposes. These included aggressively seeking public funds to "diversify the funding base," which would otherwise be borne by the system; to bring partners into the program; and to expand by "controlled growth," accepting more patients only as resources allowed, rather than by "overgrowth," mushrooming beyond available external resources.

The other members of the coalition were the state nurses' foundation, the city's public hospital and county health department, and the local health centers and drug and alcohol recovery centers. All hoped to improve their chances for getting public funds as a coalition rather than as competitors. Their success came in the formation of Mobile Services, in which they became service sites entitled to the federally paid-for servicing by the mobile unit, expanded their client base, and became members of the service's advisory committee.

Development Issues

Ethics

As a religious-based organization, the St. Francis System had to face the same reproductive and sex-related issues as the Christian Council. Its board, while it would not allow the distribution of birth control products in its own outreach services, would allow education on all birth control methods and on abortion. It also offered condoms as protection against AIDS, and educated clients about safe sex practices. While some board members "believed that the Bible said that homosexuality is immoral and that sex is sacred," the Sisters held that, "It is not our task to judge others." This position paved the way for coalition-building and grant-getting, with the first monies arriving in 1988.

Parent Support

The expansion of Mobile Services with its new external funds and coalition partners was further supported by the services of its parent, St. Francis Health System. These ranged from administrative funds and discounted administrative services to the foundation's successful campaign to establish a $1.25 million endowment for outreach services and the Healthmobile. The mobile system could draw on the information technology expertise and purchasing power of the system's hospitals. Mobile Services also had access to the grant-searching and grant-writing skills of the foundation.

Budget Building

Led by Mobile Services, the outreach services of St. Francis Health System had diversified its funding base so that the system was contributing less than 20 percent of Mobile Services' budget. Federal funds for the homeless and HIV services accounted for almost half the total, and state AIDS, immunization, and substance abuse grants covered almost another fourth of the costs, which averaged $50 a visit. All physician services, in the form of off-site backup for the direct care provided by salaried nurse practitioners, were donated. They amounted to $12,000–$13,000 per year, valued at $100 an hour. Nurses also volunteered additional services, about twice as much time, valued at about $18 an hour. And lay people contributed their time, equal to volunteer doctors' and nurses' combined, and valued at $7 an hour.

The Mobile Services' burden on St. Francis System finances was lessening, and its value to the corporate body was increasing. The Services' uniqueness as one of a handful of such programs in the country, and one of even fewer using mobile IT, was giving it and its parent national exposure. This was further incentive for the corporate family's support in the form of planning and marketing. A videotape of the service was made, and a corporate commitment was made to new "hard money" (non-grant-supported) personnel slots, and for the first time, a $50,000 contribution to capital expenditures. This was to buy the hardware and software that would tie together the mobile and fixed site units of Mobile Services and Church Help Center.

Initial financing for the laptop system had been piecemeal, amounting to about $80,000–$90,000 over about five years. Most of this was funded through the flexibility allowed in some federal grants for innovations to track clients and develop quality assurance systems in the provision of services to homeless people. It was clear that there were no off-the-shelf software or turnkey systems to serve the purposes of complex, people-responsive service programs.

Return on Investment

Throughout the process of strategic change within the St. Francis Health System and the attempt to open up health services to the poor on the streets of Southcity, the IT system at Mobile Services came to be seen as playing numerous roles, beyond the obvious and conventional one of maintaining patient records and reports. It brought a direct benefit to patients by taking necessary health services to them in a timely way and by putting them in contact with other needed services, if only by informing them about the best available source. It preserved more of the time of health services staff for providing care rather than record keeping and minimized the number of necessary clerical staff in the program's budget. By immediate reporting of scheduling and the volume of patients encountered at the 80 sites on a daily basis, the scheduling of site visits could also be tailored to changes in the movement of the people seeking services.

The laptop system could be used as a training tool for staff too, for new health professionals who had never been exposed to electronically linked mobile services, and for other units and organizations that could produce similar service programs. This also brought the potential to license the system commercially once it was refined.

Perhaps the most important value of the IT system to the corporate body was a strategic one. With public exposure, it brought a progressive and innovative image to St. Francis, serving a promotion and marketing function for both Mobile Services and St. Francis and thereby improving chances for attracting grant funds. A system called HEALTH-CHEC made accounting for and reporting expenditures to Mobile Services' ten grantors easier, quicker, and more accurate despite the diverse reporting formats. It also documented the community and patient needs that were not being addressed, further justifying more grant funds. It seemed ideal for a "shoot-from-the-hip organization," one that attempted to respond to health care needs and to the opportunities for financing those needs quickly, accurately, and attractively. As the Mobile director noted, "This (information technology) system makes us expert at being ready."

The Near Future

The new funds to upgrade the electronic system and tie it to its parent and sister units would enhance its program and strategic value, and in time, allow it to promote further direct electronic mail links to Southcity's United Way and other service agencies. Mobile Services counseled greater use of CHEC's potential by United Way, and viewed the lack of infrastructure—wiring, telephone lines, modems, and technical support—as barriers to its own closer ties with community service groups.

Capacity-building in the form of IT development, staff training, and public education was part of strategic planning for the outreach corporation. Steps were taken to develop joint ventures in service delivery and to more actively advocate for support for further services to disadvantaged people from state and federal policymakers. One newly created venture was established with Mainstreet Presbyterian Church, also a board member and electronic partner in the Church Help Center. Mobile Services would provide clinical services at Mainstreet's site, and set up a satellite facility that would include expanded laboratory and prescription drug services to supplement the mobile program, under the overall administrative and social support services of the church.

Mobile Services' electronic net would have a place in the corporation's advocacy efforts too, supplying information, preparing graphics material, educating the board and staff members who would contact policymakers, and linking partner organizations. Success would not only bring more services to more of Southcity's homeless and poor children and adults. It would also help stem the deficit in St. Francis' budget that inevitably resulted from caring for poor people, whose costs of care were higher than others' and whose sources of payment were limited or nonexistent. And, as health care reform moved toward supporting systems of managed care combined with community-oriented services, Mobile Services' community-focused IT would make it "expert at being ready."

Summary: Contexts, Conflicts, Resolutions

That "things are not as they should be" was the sense that impelled the search for new ways to do the rapidly expanding work of supporting the social outcasts of Southcity by its downtown mainline churches. Southcity experienced growing economic gaps between rich and poor, between the elite and the homeless, and between races. Comparatively few public funds supported education, medical care, and crime control, while economic expansion denuded the city of much of its older housing stock and neighborhood businesses. As the traditional task of "helping the poor" grew larger for church and community agencies, their budgets and effectiveness met obvious limits, and they looked for new sources of funds and new models of efficiency and effectiveness to justify their efforts to their donors.

Pushed by the financing imperative combined with the moral mission of some leaders, the churches worked to unify their disparate efforts. First they united their downtown works at the Church Help Center, predicated on the notion that as a coalition they would be in a better position to obtain outside funds. Then they agreed to create ties through the interagency electronic network, the Clearinghouse for Emergency Aid to the Community (CHEC). The vision was derived from Sister Marie's 1960s street-level networking and from current examples of effective business uses of IT. CHEC was intended to connect an information base on all significant programs of every public and voluntary agency to subscribing agencies in the metropolitan area. It was to be a communications and collaboration service, a common database of clients for referral, recording, delineating unmet needs, and reporting results and costs.

But other moral-religious imperatives, such as allowing gay organizations to be part of the network or providing birth control services to single women, restricted full fruition of the vision. The conflict over sharing client data was ostensibly focused on privacy, but it also protected the territorial control of each agency over its clientele, who were the basic justification for funds from church and community contributors. Another impediment to collaboration among these nonprofit groups was competition over sharing the rewards of success. In dollar terms, success could mean publicity, which would bring an improved image for grant-getting efforts and the recruitment of new donors.

There was a high price to continuing to build CHEC network. It meant breaking away from the parent Council of Churches and its core funds, as well as the initial IT system and databases. But the new parent organization for CHEC, the Church Help Center, was able to find grounds for compromise among its fewer collaborating churches. No one group imposed its own point of view. Some fundamentalist and Catholic churches, for example, believed it was not their task to judge others' behavior—a view that each previously had neither the opportunity, the necessity, nor the will to take as separate organizations pursuing their own traditional programs.

The Church Help Center obtained a sound funding base with the help of CHEC data showing its early achievements and unmet community needs, and through its active network of strategic contacts informing it of local and other resources. The center could then operate without requiring administrative expenses to be met by its member organizations. Thus, the material costs of sponsoring CHEC were small in view of expected gains for each participating church and agency. Having to rely on many sources of public, private, local, and federal funds, however, meant that large amounts of staff time had to be spent to meet grantor demands for reporting and renewal of funds.

The center's bare bones budget also demanded unpaid time from staff, especially for resetting the IT system, programming, training, monitoring, and retraining the staff or volunteers at small churches and agencies. Bargaining with vendors for computers and modems with the implicit promise of favorable publicity and potential future customers was an additional task.

The deliberate step-by-step pace of the new CHEC system's development drew in prospective user agencies and supported them with help from written, on-line, on-site, and telephone troubleshooting. Even so, the hardware was not usable when some willing participants were not able to either get an additional dedicated telephone line for CHEC or pay for the rewiring of old facilities to make them usable for CHEC.

Much of the reservoir of goodwill within the center staff came from the simple personal commitment of individuals to their own religious and social values. There were also others whose personal values were pecuniary and parasitic, and deterred CHEC's development. However, without the core administrative funding to set up and staff the center, the energies of individuals, regardless of their intentions, would have had nowhere to go in developing community IT.

There were continuing threats to network unity. Staff turnover was high at the sites requiring retraining about CHEC. Organizations were possessive of their data. And sometimes organizations placed their own priorities first when they saw that developing their own "CHEC" might bring them greater publicity and grant-getting benefits, as occurred with the homeless task force.

St. Francis

As one of the subscribers to CHEC's 450-agency database, St. Francis Mobile Health Program developed a variant of community IT by programming a laptop system and Healthmobile to "take health care to the curbside" at dozens of churches, housing shelters, soup kitchens, and open spaces where homeless people gathered.

The mobile program itself was the fusion of the personal, voluntary service of the St. Francis Hospital staff and the moral *real-politik* of the Sisters of St. Francis Health System, Inc. The corporation formed during the 1980s to maximize new financing streams and minimize uncompensated health care while preserving its century-long mission to "help the poor." The demand for unpaid care grew, and the mobile voluntary health service demonstrated a useful service and a way of keeping some patients out of the hospitals' emergency rooms, where costs of care were high. The service also presented an inspiring public image.

Mobile Services was soon incorporated by its parent system, and was charged with seeking public funds beyond the system's core financing and collaborating with other health groups to improve grant-getting. The subsequent coalition, composed mainly of public and community health agencies, had little to lose by the joint venture—they made no budget commitments. But there was much to gain, as each was caught in a budget crunch caused by cutbacks in funds and the demands of new clients—children, AIDS victims, and substance abusers—who signaled the economic distress in the community. Attaching their service sites to Mobile Services soon brought in funded health care by the Healthmobile.

Mobile Services grew rapidly with the first injection of outside funds from state, federal, and foundation grants. The enlarged program became the impetus for customizing laptop software (HEALTH) to track the work done at 80 sites. Rotating health care teams provided care to patients who might receive a service only once a year and who had many problems besides medical ones. There were no off-the-shelf programs for such complex, people-responsive services. HEALTH and CHEC, in the eyes of the service, became "everything you need to help a patient."

For St. Francis, Inc., the moral questions that plagued the Council of Churches were resolved in a similar way, by allowing all forms of education and information for all health problems, except the distribution of female birth control methods and the direct provision of abortion services. Condoms were allowed as a means to prevent the spread of AIDS. But these developments were possible only because the organizational problem of servicing new demands for care were backed up by the parent group's core administrative support, including staffing, IT expertise, wholesale rate purchasing power, preformed links to friendly suppliers, and grant-getting and public relations support—all meshing with the expertise of the new administrators recruited by the system. Again, previous experience, current need, organizational backup with funds, expertise, and useful contacts produced a workable form of community IT. Further development of the IT system became assured as it proved not only efficient and effective, but also a leading feature for image-making for the Mobile Service and the St. Francis Health System, and a resource for further IT development throughout the system.

References

American Public Health Association (APHA). 1992. *Public Health Report Card*. Washington, DC: APHA.

Bureau of the Census. 1988. *County and City Data Book*. Washington, DC: Department of Commerce.

Milio, N. 1993. "National Health Insurance: Implications for Nursing." In *Nursing Issues in the 1990s*, edited by M. Fishbein and O. Strickland. New York: Delmar.

CHAPTER

9

ELDERS IN ACTION

Using Information Technology with Young and Old in Midcity

AN ELECTRONIC net needs a social net to give it birth and sustain its berth in community life. Hard technology needs soft technology. The local community, woven from disparate threads, becomes a recognizable pattern when a few people envision new possibilities, discern a pattern, and see new ways to solve the problems they face. At least, so it seemed to the people at Friends House in Midcity's Northside district. Joining the forces of change that were affecting their lives, a few retirees at Friends wove a set of community information technology (IT) programs into Northside that would allow others, from children to institution-bound elders, to change their lives.

The City

A Strained Economy

Midcity is very middle-American. Located in the nation's heartland, its roughly 340,000 residents earned the average American household income in the early 1990s. And, like other Americans, real wages, especially from the principle manufacturing employer in the city, were growing only slowly, if at all. Many people were out of work, and others worried about their fate. Almost a tidal wave of 150 free grocery centers, sponsored by community agencies, covered the city, a fivefold increase from the early eighties. Homeowners became renters. An "impoverished middle class" emerged. As elsewhere, signs of a growing economic gap appeared as new homes, selling for more than a quarter-million dollars, were built in outlying housing estates, for "the doctors" ("Trapped" 1991).

If Midcity was typical of middle-class, urban America, it was part of a state that was not. State support for many services was below national norms, including access to basic health care, education, public health services, and safe drinking water, while rates of violent crime, child poverty, and unemployment were high (APHA 1992).

Changing Populations

So a thread of social change, connecting the national economy, corporate downsizing, fewer good-paying jobs, joblessness, and child poverty, came through the lives of the people of Midcity's Northside district. There, young, lower-income families lived among older, middle-income retirees in large converted single family dwellings reminiscent of an affluent and genteel past. The children were dropping out of school; young mothers needed paying jobs; and older people were retiring with their career skills, energy, and health in good order, and with time at their disposal. These too were trendlines that stretched across urban America (GAO 1992a, 1992b).

A Nucleus for Renewal

In the middle of Northside was church-sponsored Friends House. It followed the revived settlement house tradition of the heartland, which began in the sixties when many church congregations joined the "white flight" to the suburbs, leaving "urban ministries" to address the growing problems of inner cities. The Friends House was staff-designed in the seventies to be useful and durable. It was large and flat, esthetic in its simplicity, bright, cleanable, and economical, but without windows—a newer tradition arising from the urban riots of the previous decade.

Initiated and led by a board from five mainline Protestant denominations, more recently adding neighborhood residents, smaller sects, and Catholic churches, Friends was a "ministry of Christian caring that seeks resources to help resolve the problems of the socially, spiritually, physically, and economically depressed . . . your family in the heart of the city." It explained its philosophy by appropriating the biblical story of feeding 5,000 people with a boy's two fishes and five loaves:

> Others (in the crowd of 5,000) who had resources but had not disclosed them, began to feel compelled to share. As more people were willing to share the little they had, others revealed what they had hidden for themselves in their satchels and pouches. As a result of this collective food, there was more than enough to go around for everybody. This kind of miracle is what is needed to bring the injustice of hunger to an end.

Conventional Services and Problems

Among the Friends programs was a Food Pantry that supplied about 30,000 meals a year. There were also emergency rental and utilities funds—until the funds ran out before the end of each fiscal year. There was an after-school program of arts, crafts, music, dance, and Spanish classes; field activities for young children and teens; clubs for single mothers and older adults, and a large recruitment program for retiree volunteers to use their skills for other community service groups, engaging several hundred elders a year.

This rather typical social service menu—which in fact captured only about a third of its $400,000 budget—was one part of a longer-term effort, which included Friends' initiating and staffing the Northside Planning Task Force through its neighborhood development efforts. It brought together city and business leaders to integrate the north side into the city's downtown redevelopment scheme for both housing and commercial development. Other outreach programs and intergroup work took up about half the budget. Most of the staff of 10 to 12 full and part-time men and women focused on guiding, coordinating, and training volunteers to lead the array of activities, whether supervising day camp, teaching teens about AIDS, or planting trees in the neighborhood.

"I'm sorry but we're out of funds for the month" was a frequent response to callers and drop-in seekers of emergency aid, people who needed money for rent or overdue bills until the next paycheck. Budgeting was an increasing problem throughout the 1980s and well into the 1990s. There were more people in greater need, with bleaker futures, while all sources of budget funds were being cut: the quarter that came from government grants, the third given by the United Way, the third donated by the 60 sponsoring churches and individual contributors.

City funds in recent years were shifted to crime control at the expense of emergency assistance; charitable giving was less generous in the slowing economy, and the mainline churches were more wary about giving funds to their national headquarters, which traditionally was the source of "home missions" funding like Friends House.

New Directions from the Old

A changing economy, a changing population, and an all too common "crunch" between resources and needs impelled a search for new ways for Friends to do its work. Yet another thread of change reached Friends House in the later eighties. In an effort to conserve staff time, Friends got a computer for word processing and bookkeeping, along with an "expert" who volunteered to set up and keep their accounts. Without warning, she "took off under mysterious circumstances," in the euphemistic terms of the elderly minister and longtime director. She left no documentation of the computer programs, leaving Friends fiscally and technologically confused.

It happened that a board member—a grandmother and retired math teacher who had earned a graduate degree in computer science at age 65—volunteered to "troubleshoot the system." She accomplished the task and stayed to pick up on the technological interest that began to change the face of Friends House and its interface with the community. "We could not have done any of this without her," reported the Director.

The Electronic Environment

Friends House's 70-year-old computer expert became a linchpin connecting other more subtle and pervasive movement toward IT from Midcity leaders. The local school board, in a district that had admittedly been slower than most in IT, had just committed an unprecedented $3 million for new computers and teacher training to support computer work from kindergarten through twelfth grade. The city's museum also set up a hands-on computer technology center.

Then came a new citywide electronic network, Freenet, unique because of its nonuniversity origin and rapidly gaining popularity since its inception in 1989. It was begun by local businesses and technology firms, the library and state bar associations, and local press, led by none other than a member of the Friends board. The sponsoring businesses not only contributed the hardware, but also supplied most of the $55,000 annual operating funds for its 1.5 staff. These donations were tax-deductible and would promote a wider market for their electronic products and services. But the greater value may well have been in public relations at a time when these leading national firms were cutting back on their local work forces.

An Open Network

Freenet was to become a ready supporter and collaborator with Friends' IT programs. It was based in free-use offices at the private Heartland University, and like other Freenets, it was free to all users who had access to computers with a modem. With a grant from the state legislature, Freenet provided public access computers in all 30 of Midcity's public libraries, in government buildings, and in community agencies in its tri-county area. There, people could access a vast array of information, including government and business data and services, legal and medical help, elder and other social service resources, and education, youth, and library programs, each with question-answer and open forum modules for discussion and feedback. Through Freenet, users could also access other Freenets and a few catalogs from university libraries in other states. The most used service was the state's job service listing for job seekers.

Before Freenet's registered users reached 6,000 in the early nineties, its public access computers were being set up with a training service by volunteers from the new Friends Seniors Computer Club.

Community IT: Necessity, Opportunity, and Invention

The relentless need for new funds, the growing presence of information technologies, and the place of the Friends director on the advisory board of Midcity's federally funded community development block grant program came together in a new idea. Friends House sought block grant funds in 1989 for a computer learning center to expand its after-school program, steered by its new elderly IT expert, who said, "Our life is going to be built around computers. . . . For these (neighborhood) kids to be employable, they've got to know computers. . . . They are beginning to get a little in the schools. . . . Besides, teaching computers is just another approach to the informal education that Friends has always done . . . and it helps us, our staff, get into the computer world."

The Computer Learning Center

The grant of $12,000 was awarded at the start of the 1990s. The new center was for children and "as many others as possible." Within months it had a full schedule of classes for children from preschool age to teens, for single mothers wanting to learn job skills and other adults, and for seniors—children's lab, career lab, neighborhood lab, senior lab—and an open lab for anyone who wished to use the equipment, all supervised by trained volunteers.

The software ranged from age-graded programs for basic literacy skills to natural and social science, health and "life skills," and computer skills, such as spreadsheets, databases, and desktop publishing. The volunteer tutors, who were recruited and trained by the center, were mainly retired teachers, a women's auxiliary from the sponsoring churches, and members of Friends House's own Seniors Computer Club. Overall coordination came from the Friends in-house IT expert. Within two years, about 250 children from the neighborhood were using the center about once a week, as were 40 seniors and 10 single mothers, shepherded by a core of 18 volunteers scheduled throughout the week.

Getting the Technology

Setting up the learning center was akin to making five loaves and two fishes feed a multitude. The Friends board formed a computer committee headed by a minister–computer buff. He recruited IT experts from local firms who were also members of the Friends House sponsoring congregations. They decided to use local rather than national vendors to take advantage of close-by support services and establish longer-term relationships.

The available funds could buy only four computer systems and two printers. But by telling the local vendors that "we could of course get our hardware by mail order, but we want to deal with you," Friends got not only discounted prices but the seller's donation of two more refurbished personal computers. He gained from a tax deduction for charitable giving and good public relations.

Software that would be useful and fun for the variety of potential Friends users was beyond both the budget and experience of its in-house experts. But the local public school IT coordinator supplied ongoing guidance and gave the center "shareware" programs, the noncommercial software offerings that are available on many electronic networks from individual programmers. Within a year Friends' own senior citizens too were downloading selected shareware from Freenet for the children's use, vastly expanding the learning center's library of available educational software.

These riches, however, created a consequent "crunch," as someone had to become proficient at each new item in order to teach it to others, and this often demanded time that was not immediately available.

SeniorNet

One other new piece of hardware was donated to the center—a "dumb" terminal and modem, capable of accessing Freenet and SeniorNet, a national electronic network for older people. The donors were five physician eye specialists, ophthalmologists who ran a local private medical practice, the Eye Center. The gift was duly labeled and publicly acknowledged, which brought four more donated terminals from other local physicians.

Distant Origins

The initial gift represented another thread to be woven into the IT fabric emerging at Friends. Its remote origins were buried in the fact that in the Medicare reforms of the 1980s, payment and indications for cataract surgery, primarily done for the elderly, had been cut back. It had been a chief source of ophthalmologists' patients and income. Fewer visits from elders, and growing numbers of competing eye specialists in the cities led these physicians to devise a variety of ways to attract more patients. Some preferred not to resort to direct advertising. They sought visibility through community involvement by sponsoring a local SeniorNet site. Of the almost 40 sites across the country in the early nineties, almost half were sponsored by ophthalmologists. The physicians from Midcity first learned about this form of community service, which could also attract elderly patients to their office practice, at an eye specialists' conference.

The general focus of SeniorNet, a nonprofit organization begun in the 1980s, was to "bring wisdom to the information age" by teaching computer skills to older adults through locally sponsored sites where classes were offered in computer applications and through low-cost on-line electronic services. There were about 4,000 SeniorNet members in the early nineties (SeniorNet 1992).

The SeniorNet site in Midcity was unique because it was not a physical site. Its classes were taught in facilities and on computers provided by Heartland University. The university was also searching for ways to interest elders in its own programs as it attempted to widen its educational offerings to meet ever-growing budget needs.

The lack of a site where elders could come to learn and use computers, as well as communicate on SeniorNet by electronic mail—as they could at other SeniorNet sites—may have been a hidden benefit to the community as well as to the physicians. The "site," as a matter of survival, required dispersal into community locations and reliance on community people for its development. The Eye Center specialists made a significant initial investment of about $10,000 for the first-year charges and costs to the national SeniorNet organization, and they provided about 10 to 15 percent of their public relations director's time to coordinate the site program, mainly for setting up computer classes.

It happened that the first SeniorNet computer class taught at the university included the just-retired director of Friends House, fresh from suffering the pangs of deciphering Friends' computerized bookkeeping problem. Having bought a personal computer, he wanted to extend his retirement career through Freenet and SeniorNet. He was immediately recruited to join the Eye Center's newly created SeniorNet steering committee, to develop the program and entice seniors into the courses and into volunteering as instructors in the university classrooms.

The Seniors Computer Club

Back at Friends, the newly opened computer learning center was teaching elders; and so began the Friends Seniors Computer Club. Initially, Friends went to Freenet and obtained a list of the 60 elderly users as a source for recruiting the first students and future volunteer lab staff. They then became, after a training and supervisory period, instructors for the children's classes, with a little extra guidance and support for dealing with the occasional frustrations of dealing with energetic youngsters.

By early collaborative planning, SeniorNet and Friends developed complementary programs. SeniorNet provided structured classes limited to seven-week one-day sessions about twice a year, while Friends House's labs and club, available year-round, provided a practice site as well a place to use Freenet, get introduced to new software, help other seniors, and staff or teach the other labs in the learning center.

The center was a safe place for novices to learn at their own pace. "They are very brave [elderly] people that sit down and look at this machine." Some require more time than others to become friends with "the machine," but as one member put it, "Who's going to take the time to help them, if not us (at Friends House)? . . . Besides, out of this comes a lot of fun and fellowship . . . an opportunity to share . . . we sort of have a rotation of seniors; as they learn, they teach others . . . we find the more you help people with problems, the more they help you, and you learn also."

Friends and SeniorNet promoted each other's programs, and shared committee members, instructors, and community events, like the annual potluck supper and the local SeniorNet conference open to all on its 900 person mailing list. Most participants were between 60 and 75 years old, middle-income, well-educated, healthy elders who usually wanted to learn about computers so they could connect better with their grandchildren and "keep up with the times." SeniorNet classes were fully enrolled, "graduating" 150 elders in a "semester." Meanwhile, Friends was expanding its senior resources, pointing to still more program development in the community.

Electronic Sharing

Another original student at the Heartland SeniorNet classes was a retired industrial engineer who wanted to be conversant with his computer-teaching daughter. He "got hooked" and joined the Seniors Computer Club at Friends and was also asked to join the SeniorNet steering committee. The germ of a new joint venture was a request by a local nursing home to set up a computer donated by a family who had used it to access home care support for the mother with Alzheimer's Disease. Having once accomplished that task, which included programming the nursing home's calendar of events, patient preference files, and kitchen inventory, the steering committee agreed to set up other computers that had been donated to Friends, and to solicit more computers for other community sites such as nursing homes, retirement housing, and social service agencies. Friends' seniors offered to do the training on site, and the SeniorNet sponsoring physicians supplied free modems after the university determined whether the systems were working properly.

Electronic links with elders were added to Freenet in new modules called Senior Citizens and Friends Electronic Pen Pals, aimed especially at people in nursing homes or otherwise homebound citizens. Several hundred messages were on this medium at any given time. Few Midcity seniors used the national SeniorNet on-line system, costing about $10 a month after the $25 annual membership fee: "Why subscribe to SeniorNet when Freenet is free?"

Additional reaching out with classes and placement of computers in nursing homes was to be limited in the foreseeable future because of the lack of volunteer staff to conduct the activities. SeniorNet sites elsewhere in the country, having a physical center, had somewhat more staff time allocated to program activity, but were not undertaking such outreach ventures.

A Satellite Center

Friends Computer Learning Center soon developed a clone through its Northside redevelopment work in a program at a public housing site where a boys and girls club was activated under grant funds. With a special grant from United Way and a modem from SeniorNet, Friends set up a lab, supplying the organization and training by its elder volunteers. The dream was for both learning centers to have multimedia educational systems, combining color, interactive sound, image, text, and data to draw students into the fascination of new worlds of information and education.

The Future

Another dream at Friends House was a career skills program to join local small businesses, people who wanted to develop job and enterprise skills, and the computer learning center. This would make possible usable skills and job placements benefiting both job seekers and the small business people who needed skilled workers but could not afford the few that were available.

But dreams were kept for the future, as Friends sought in the first years of the nineties to meet its budget deficits within the gloomy context of Midcity's and the nation's economy. It applied for grant funds cautiously—a task demanding staff time and grant-getting skills—while cultivating its traditional base of support in the mainstream denominations, not wanting to alienate them. It refined this local source by expanding its board to smaller, neighborhood denominations and sects, as well as to the Catholic churches. And, rather than going to the central church structures, it began to take its message, its record of invention and extension, directly to the congregations, seeking funds and volunteers.

Through its board members, Friends also went more often to Midcity businesses, which had proved responsive at least to ad hoc requests for computer-related resources, ranging from expertise to hardware, especially once the learning center was in operation. Recycling computers offered the possibility of a renewable resource, but it was an unorganized and time-demanding task for the future.

Summary: Conditions, Issues, Solutions

Tight national and local economies brought a fiscal resource crunch to public and private funders who mandated graphic results from funded programs, while there were growing needs in the community for Friends House's neighborhood services. This situation led Friends to search for new resources and new ways to do its work. At the same time, a new and growing fund of experience, energy, interest in learning, and the time to do it was waiting in the accumulated wealth of experience of a retired citizenry. Midcity's schools and other institutions, and the private sector, were bent on developing information technology to improve their efficiency and to prepare a work force and polity to strengthen the economy and community life.

Friends House's long-standing as a community institution had cast a dense net of social connections, allowing it to learn about and be involved in new developments. These included the tri-county electronic Freenet, open to public users through widely placed public computer terminals, and SeniorNet, itself a local venture by private ophthalmologists and the university to attract elderly clientele. All the contributors to these IT ventures hoped in some way to sustain their professional, public, or corporate markets and advance their image as reliable local producers. With these events creating an enabling climate, Friends House's elderly leaders drew on its organizational contacts for information about new federal grants, IT expertise, and discounted IT equipment. Friends combined these with the human resources of its senior volunteers to do in new ways what it had always done: support children and families in their quest for a better life—the task that justified its existence to its donors.

Using its organizational net to its church donors, whose members knew IT experts, and the public schools, which could advise on low-cost software, Friends Learning Center expanded beyond the time available to train volunteers to staff it; there was always a resource crunch between attending to immediate center services and training new volunteers to assist with them.

One resource that it had was its good name and the trust that its youthful and elderly clientele had in it. This it could bestow on donors, thereby acquiring new hardware, including equipment to access SeniorNet. Friends and SeniorNet, each aware of its own resource limits, also recognized that collaboration could be a win-win venture. They thus shared sites, programs, volunteer staff, and clientele, and both grew as a result of bartering and visibility. Communication was further improved by cross-membership on advisory boards, mutual public membership meetings, and joint planning to avoid schedule conflicts.

Friends House's joint ventures made possible further electronic and program outreach to elders in nursing homes, others on Freenet, and children in another neighborhood center. But, as always, goodwill by the volunteers was not enough to match the need without further material support in the form of trainers, equipment, and technical assistance.

To shape its future in ways that would meet economic, social, and technological demands, Friends was attempting to broaden its resource base by expanding its board beyond mainline denominations, taking its achievements to local congregations instead of church hierarchies, and seeking to recycle discarded computer hardware and software from firms that wanted a friendly local face. All of this required staff time to plan, initiate, and organize. Again, enough material help to sustain sound development often seemed just beyond reach.

Changes in the economy, in people, in technology, and in the relations among organizations and groups came together at Friends House, a place with a mission and a compelling set of problems about its future. It recognized the new environment and began to use it to reinvent its future, relying in large measure on the time, energy, and commitment of the old.

References

American Public Health Association (APHA). 1992. *Public Health Report Card.* Washington, DC: APHA.

General Accounting Office (GAO). 1992a. Education Issues. Washington, DC: U.S. Congress, December.

———. 1992b. Housing Issues. Washington, DC: U.S. Congress, December.

SeniorNet. 1992. *Bringing a SeniorNet Site to Your Community.* San Francisco: SeniorNet.

"Trapped in the Impoverished Middle Class." 1991. *New York Times*, 17 November, 1.

SECTION C

Distance Work and Distance Learning

If every tool could perform its own work when ordered, or by seeing what to do in advance . . . If thus shuttles wove and quills played harps of themselves, master-craftsmen would have no need of assistants and masters no need of slaves.

Aristotle, *Politics, Book I*

. . . changes in the (information) infrastructure are likely to broaden the gap between those who can access communication services and use information strategically, and those who cannot. . . . the people most likely to be adversely affected are those whom the new . . . technologies could help the most—the poor, the educationally disadvantaged, the geographically and technologically isolated, and the struggling small and medium-sized business.

Office of Technology Assessment, U.S. Congress, *Critical Connections*, 1990

CHAPTER

10

INFORMATION TECHNOLOGY FOR EDUCATION AND ECONOMIC ENTERPRISE

ONCE UPON a time in the first Industrial Revolution, home workers were the piece-rate workers who sewed and knitted in their houses for clothing manufacturers. Over the decades, writers and illustrators joined the ranks of home workers. Now there are about 35 million home workers of whom one in ten have regular office-based jobs but do some work at home (Dixon 1991). As the new information technologies (IT) create new patterns of economic production, new forms of off-site "distance work" are evolving in homes and local IT centers to meet social as well as economic imperatives. These new forms are creating bridges between work, education, and home, bringing together information, IT services, and users.

Rapid changes in employment and social patterns suggest the need for dual and multipurpose IT centers responsive to local community needs. The growing number of poor school children in rural areas, especially among minorities and in isolated, underfunded school systems, makes "distance learning" between school systems as attractive an option as distance work is becoming to employers (GAO 1994b). With new immigrants, single parents, and job seekers at all ages, life-long learning for all social groups has become necessary to enable people to participate in their communities as income earners and citizens.

The business community learned the importance of designing IT support systems by involving users. Both employees and customers report a better quality of life when technical assistance and other supports are ongoing and attuned to their needs. This supportive infrastructure includes physical requisites—space, equipment, wiring—and human resources—skilled trainers and troubleshooters (Kling 1992). Some countries, like Norway, require worker involvement in the design of such systems (Schneider and Ciborra 1983).

Large firms also acknowledge the benefits of using IT to advance their personnel with ongoing training and development. One coalition organized the National Technical University in the late eighties. It now offers over 450 courses by satellite through more than 25 universities to employees at over 40 companies as part of a graduate degree program. Other industries also have their own networks, such as the Hospital Satellite Network (OTA 1989).

Yet small organizations, whether small businesses or service organizations like public school systems, cannot afford either to design or use IT systems (OTA 1989; Kling and Dunlop 1993).

The Economic Push

The Beginnings

In the 1960s, a freelance systems analyst, impelled as a working mother-to-be, organized a group of similarly situated women software developers into an enterprise now employing over 1,000 people who work from their home-based computers. Distance work was made easier for some of these freelancers by electronically linked local work centers with computer work stations where they could work very close to their homes. This new form of home and local center-based distance work, made possible by IT, has since developed into more elaborate variations. Known as "telework"—sending work electronically to the worker instead of sending the worker to work—the term first came into use in this country in the 1970s (Nilles et al. 1976).

A companion concept, defined as center-based interactive IT for information and education, was demonstrated in the later seventies. Supported by local government, using two-way cable television, it "offered to the community the best possible educational and informational programs." These programs were organized and produced by community volunteers, fed into the local cable system, and delivered to local sites, such as a community center or senior center, and as a regular subscriber channel to homes (Burns 1981a,b). In contrast to larger commercial regional or national interactive formats, this center-based system used television as a live, two-way medium that depended on verbal audience participation and feedback. For example, through a series of national issues forums, it raised relevant issues, such as the day care dilemma and drug crisis, while encouraging home viewers and the studio audience to actively take part in the discussion. Community agencies such as the chamber of commerce, county bar association, and hospitals used the system to conduct their outreach, information, and referral services (OTA 1991).

Joining these telework and community education initiatives in the eighties, dozens of remote and rural towns, first in Scandinavia and then in Europe, began to develop "electronic town halls" ("telehouses" or "community teleservice centers"), as the next case will depict. These allowed not only communal viewing, but also, in various combinations and alternative sites, video and computer conferencing, videotex, telefax, mobile terminals, training and education with and about IT, collective siting of work stations for distance work in commerce, health, and social welfare, and public information and meeting facilities (Qvortrup 1992).

The Nineties

The development of local IT centers in the 1990s seems to be forging two paths, one commercial and economic, the other education and community oriented, in response to the priorities and financial requirements of particular environments. The most extensive uses of IT centers in the United States have followed the enterprise route, with the West Coast leading the way.

The L.A. County Test

In the late eighties, Los Angeles County employed 80,000 people in 39 departments responsible for a population greater than 42 of the states, and covering a space the size of Delaware and Rhode Island combined. It faced both the pervasive realities of the changing American work force, to which most major businesses were responding, and the specific imperatives of California that forced new thinking about how to redesign and retain an efficient employee base (GAO 1994a).

The majority of American workers have jobs that involve information processing—and are therefore portable. A continuously growing share of employees are women, and typical families are dual career or single parent households with attendant work-home stresses showing up in large increases in absenteeism and workers' compensation claims.

In L.A. County, in addition to opening on-site child care centers and offering flexible benefits programs, more was needed to accommodate severe state and federal budget cutbacks, the limitations of the no-property-tax Proposition 13, and the unaffordability of local housing, sometimes requiring employees to commute over 200 miles round trip. The state also mandated reduced work trips by government employees to control air pollution and cut down on traffic delays that cost a half-million dollars a year in lost work time (Dixon 1991).

Telecommuting was chosen to address this daunting, but not unique, set of employer issues. Within two years 2,500 workers from most of the county's 250 job classifications (e.g., planning and contract monitoring, health, social, and in-home support services) were teleworkers. They did some of their work through computers from their homes or from satellite IT-equipped offices based in local health centers, libraries, and elsewhere. Based on a similar pilot program conducted by state employees working two to three days at home, the cost savings per worker each year were expected to be about $8,000 in productivity, recruitment and training, absenteeism, office space, and parking costs (Pitzer 1991; Brain and Page 1991a).

In any case, the growing program was seen as a success by workers and managers as well as by other communities that modeled neighborhood IT work centers after the county program (Drummer 1991; Hulett 1991). To spur further changes in both public and private enterprise, a new state law allocated some of the gasoline tax to match half the annual cost (up to $1,000 per worker) of creating telecommuting employees (O'Connor 1991).

The Hawaiian Demonstration

A variation and still more extensive effort in center-based telecommuting began in Oahu, the main island of Hawaii, as part of an overall transportation plan to reduce traffic congestion (SMS Research 1991). Begun in 1989, the Telework Center Demonstration Project was a state response to some special problems beyond the budgetary, pollution, and workforce issues faced by most governments. Hawaii had the lowest employment rates of the states and least access to U.S. employment markets, as well as very high land and business costs and gasoline prices. Further, many residents were on remote islands and seeking the same kinds of opportunities as others on more developed islands.

Initiated with U.S. Department of Transportation support and a public-private task force of government, higher education, and IT industry representatives, a center was developed in an Oahu suburb. The state contributed a fifth of the total costs, which included a center facilitator, and companies added almost a half-million dollars in mainly in-kind contributions of personnel and equipment. The center provided office space, shared use of equipment, access to government databases, and communications services. Any group could rent the office space, which was free during the demonstration. The early users included state departments such as taxation, education, judiciary, agriculture, and private firms, including banking and legal services. These groups provided customer ("front office") services and also performed internal organization ("back room") work, thus saving time and expense for employee, business, client, and citizen travel.

Employees saved about eight hours of weekly travel time, and those who worked at the center at least three days a week cut fuel use by almost half. Applied to 5 percent of the Hawaiian workforce, this would save about 8 percent of fuel consumption a year (Brain and Page 1991a). Other studies, including one done in the United Kingdom, showed that 15 percent of working days could be done by telecommuting in the mid-1990s at a savings of 16 percent of energy use per worker (British Telecommunications 1992). Beyond Hawaii's dollar benefits from travel savings and new local economic activity, a one-year evaluation showed high job satisfaction for workers and managers, higher or equal productivity compared to downtown offices, and an unexpected camaraderie among workers of the participating companies (SMS Research 1991).

Critics were concerned that such centers, if located in remote areas, might further isolate disadvantaged populations. This prospect would have to be balanced against the possibility of new job and service opportunities for those communities. The Hawaii legislature reported that almost 10 percent of the total workforce might appropriately be teleworkers within 15 years, and it proposed a tax credit of up to half the technology costs for setting up such centers throughout the islands (Brain and Page 1991b).

Euro-Variants

Some European governments, such as The Netherlands, provided more generous support for teleworking and with greater emphasis on humanitarian purposes besides relieving traffic congestion and increasing productivity (Brain and Page 1991a). To ease the worklife of the physically impaired and support workers with domestic responsibilities, the Dutch Transportation Department provided IT equipment to its home-based telecommuters. The results of the initial efforts were similar to the U.S. demonstrations in travel and other efficiencies, although the home workers did not feel that the "quality of worklife" necessarily improved. The government stressed the need for voluntary participation, phased-in development, and responsive, high-quality training and support. In this, one of the most dense and advanced of countries, teleworking will continue to expand (Jongerius, Hagenbeek, and Overmars 1991).

Scotland

In the 90 islands under the jurisdiction of the Highlands and Islands Development Board of Scotland, most of the 100,000 residents were unaware of information technology (Watt 1991). Entering the 1990s, one of the islands became a site of one of six teleservice centers in a joint venture between the board and British Telecom (BT), sharing the costs in a 30/70 split. BT, with its extensive telecommunications monopoly in the United Kingdom, was setting up telework for its telephone operators in their homes across Great Britain. It found an interest in developing an awareness of its products in remote parts of the country, while the board sought economic and community development for distant islanders (HIDB 1989).

One of the six demonstration sites of the joint $30 million investment was a community teleservice center operated by an umbrella organization for the voluntary organizations of one island community, the Council of Voluntary Services (Ogilvie and Clark 1991). It offered a range of organization support, including desktop publishing, communications, IT training, and shared hardware and software, as well as consultation in developing community-based services and small businesses. It was able to operate on about $30,000 a year, half coming from the development grant in the first three years (Islay & Jura 1991). The centers were expected to create at least 500 jobs (HIDB 1989).

Denmark

Many more local IT centers in Europe provided models for the European Union's new telecommunications infrastructure development program, supported with $45 billion over a ten-year period. Combining enterprise and education for adults, an urban center in Denmark, for example, offered self-serve, customer, and consultative IT services to small businesses, and offered a range of training programs with and about IT to public agencies, such as the city's employment office and local employers, and multimedia educational programs for the Ministry of Social Welfare. These services made for a profit-making venture, with income of over $300,000 annually (Ipsen 1990).

Scandinavia

Following the lead of Sweden and Denmark, which are described in the next chapter, Finland and Norway experimented with over 120 variants of IT centers in the last decade, in forms "somewhere between a coffeehouse and a post office" (Qvortrup 1992; Kristiansen and Blom 1988). An emerging consensus is that in order to operate within budget or at a profit, the centers have to be responsive to local needs but also networked in a cooperative relationship with other centers.

Education in and for Communities

Distance learning means transporting information, not people, through technology. A third of U.S. schoolchildren are poorly educated because of shortages of staff and resources in small, isolated schools. Remote learning through IT could bring skilled teachers of science, mathematics, foreign languages, and health to these sites (OTA 1989).

In spite of its benefits, this form of learning can also reinforce students' feeling of isolation if IT is overused—just as IT monitoring at workplaces can lower staff performance if abused (OTA 1989; Grant and Higgins 1991). Thus, the importance of collaborative and locally attuned design, of an appropriate balance and calibration of both physical and human resources.

Open Learning Centers Network

There is a regional-cluster design among the more than 35 sites of the Open Learning Centers Network in the Texas-sized state of Queensland, Australia. With 2 million of the state's 3 million people living outside the capitol, the centers provide post-secondary education through the community college system. Around-the-clock access enables use of a full range of IT, including two-way conferencing and satellite communications, supported by government and industry funds. Regional and center-based coordinators manage the rapidly growing system, conducting training and encouraging participation and collaboration with partners in universities, schools, industry worksites, and government offices. Other states responded to local community interest with similar centers in the early 1990s, and the federal government began plans for a national system of open learning centers in this vast country of only 16 million people (Qvortrup 1992).

Council for Computers in Education

Still another design for education with IT was developed in the highly populated developing nation of Malaysia. As a means to educate and encourage the use of IT among students, and as a way to conduct public health education, the Council for Computers in Education sponsored a national competition for a series of computer-based presentations in healthy living. Collaborating with the Ministries of Education and Technology, the winning software was converted to video for use by public and educational television systems (Soon 1991).

TENET of Texas

A network designed to connect teachers and administrators statewide in a Teachers Educational Network (TENET) in the early nineties showed that most participants used TENET more than they had expected. The vast majority found it very useful, especially the communications services (rather than databases) and access to sources on the Internet, such as discussion groups. Their views of its importance to themselves, and ways to improve it, including better training and more time-saving simplifications, were similar to those expressed by other users (H.R. 1757 1993).

New Connections

In the early 1990s, new resources were coming on-line for teachers, students, and administrators. One such resource was a collaboration of several state school systems, a commercial firm, and the public access National Public Telecomputing Network (NPTN). It was developing curricular databases for teachers; information services on technology, government, science, and health; news services; and on-line simulations—all of which could be used directly in classrooms (Grundner 1993). As the national information infrastructure proliferates to local schools and worksites, such educational resources will be readily accessible to learners, trainers, and planners.

Yet, where the new wireline technologies bypass local organizations and communities, their constituents will inevitably be ever further behind their counterparts.

References

Brain, D., and A. Page. 1991a. *Review of Current Experiences and Prospects for Teleworking*. Report. Brussels, Belgium: Commission of the European Community, DG XIII, December.

———. 1991b. Telework: An Alternate Route to the Work Place. *Hawaii Pacific Information Times 3* (9): 1.

British Telecommunications. 1992. *A Study of the Environmental Impact of Teleworking*. London: BT.

Burns, R. 1981a. "Technology is Not Enough." Presented at the American Council on Education, Washington, DC.

———. 1981b. "You Can See the Results, But What Went into the Making?" Report. New York: Alternative Media Center, New York University.

Dixon, R. 1991. *Telecommuting in Los Angeles County*. Report. Los Angeles, CA: County of Los Angeles, Chief Administrative Office, 26 August.

Drummer, R. 1991. "Avoid Gridlock by Working at Home—Via a Computer. *Daily Bulletin*, 23 June, B1.

General Accounting Office. 1994a. "Private Sector Elder Care." Washington, DC: U.S. Congress, 31 January.

———. 1994b. "Rural Children." Washington, DC: U.S. Congress, 11 January.

Grant, R., and C. Higgins. 1991. "The Impact of Computerized Performance Monitoring on Service Work." *Information Systems Research* 2 (2): 116–41.

Grundner, T. 1993. "NPTN and Ameritech to Create Online Educational Program." Internet release, 29 September.

Highlands and Islands Development Board (HIDB). 1989. "New Initiative to Put Highlands and Islands at Forefront of Communications Technology." *Top Business* (UK), November 1, 2.

H.R. 1757. 1993. *High Performance Computing and High Speed Networking Application Act of 1993*. House Subcommittee on Science, Space, and Technology. Hearings on 27 April, 6 May, and 11 May. Washington, DC: U.S. Congress, 160–75.

Hulett, S. 1991. "Telecommuting Is Off to a "Fax" Start." *California County* (May/June): 18, 26.

Ipsen, F. 1990. *DATARIET—Community Teleservice Center for an Urban Region*. Report. Vejle, Denmark, October.

Islay and Jura Council of Voluntary Service. 1991. *Community: Islay Teleservice Centre*. Report. Argyll, Scotland: Islay & Jura Council of Voluntary Service.

Jongerius, A., F. Hagenbeek, and J. Overmars. 1991. *Telecommuting R.I.V., A Department of the Ministry of Transport: Summary, Conclusions and Recommendations*. Report. Amsterdam, The Netherlands: Overmars & Partners, March.

Kling, R. 1992. "Behind the Terminal: The Critical Role of Computing Infrastructure in Effective Information Systems Development and Use." In *Challenges and Strategies for Research in Systems Development,* edited by J. Cotterman and R. Senn. New York: John Wiley, 153–201.

Kling, R., and C. Dunlop. 1993. "Controversies about Computerization and the Character of White Collar Worklife." *Informatics Society* 9: 1–29.

Kristiansen, T., and D. Blom. 1988. *The Jevnaker Project: Two Experiments with Live Interactive Television.* Report. Oslo, Norway: Norwegian Telecommunications Administration.

Nilles, J., and M. Plackett. 1976. *Telecommuting and Economic Development*. Los Angeles, CA: JALA Associates, Inc.

O'Connor, R. 1991. "Assembly Trying to Boost Work Out of Office." *The Orange County Register*, 6 June, 3.

Office of Technology Assessment (OTA). 1989. *Linking for Learning*. Washington, DC: U.S. Congress.

———. 1991. *Rural America at the Crossroads: Networking for the Future*. Washington, DC: U.S. Congress, April.

Ogilvie, M., and A. Clark. 1991. *Islay & Jura Council of Voluntary Service. Annual Report.* Argyll, Scotland: Islay & Jura Council of Voluntary Service.

Pitzer, M. 1991. "Telecommunicating Gains Popularity But Skeptics Remain." *Los Angeles Daily News*, 3 March, 4.

Qvortrup, L., ed. 1992. "Learning at a Distance." *CTSC International Newsletter*, no. 3.

Schneider, L., and C. Ciborra. 1983. *Systems Design for, with, and by Users.* New York: North-Holland.

SMS Research. 1991. *Final Evaluation Report on Year One of the Hawaii Telework Center Demonstration Project*. Honolulu, HI: Department of Transportation, State of Hawaii, 8 January.

Soon, T. 1991. Personal Communication. Malaysian Council for Computers-in-Education, Kuala Lumpur, 8 July.

Watt, J. 1991. *Community Teleservice Centres in the Highlands and Islands of Scotland: A Progress Report*. Edinburgh, Scotland: Highlands and Islands Development Board.

CHAPTER

11

BRINGING BUSINESS TO HILL PARK, UNITED KINGDOM

A Rural Community Moves Out with Information Technology

AGAINST THE familiar black-greenness of the English countryside in the northern region east of Manchester, was a slate-roofed farmhouse of the early nineteenth century. Its heritage was still visible by the words chiseled on its stone window ledges—"dairy room," "cheese room." The farmhouse and barns, renovated within the laws governing historic preservation sites, augured a new way of rural life not simply for the twentieth, but more likely for the early twenty-first century. The site was recreated as the Hill Park Telebusiness Center in 1992. It represented the view that viable communities, those that could support the social and environmental values essential to human security, must be based on sustainable economies that are information-supported and competent in producing information, regardless of where the information originates or where it is needed. Communities must become nodes in the "information society."

To roam the surrounding Hill Valley, one could see little obvious change from the stereotypical life of the countryside. Hills dotted by tiny villages of a few hundred or thousand people, neatly kept farms, and occasional mining sites and stone quarries denoting the traditional economic base of the region over decades and centuries. But this was only a surface view.

Town and Countryside

By the 1980s, fundamental, irreversible changes were occurring in country life, revealed in a study and in the words of lifelong residents in a commissioned report on the Hill Park District. The population had grown only slightly over the 1980s as young families moved away for lack of affordable housing—once available at about $25,000, but later gentrified and selling at $125,000—and ex-urban professionals moved in from nearby Sheffield. There was apparent affluence and evidence of a new phenomenon, "counterurbanization," revealed in the sentiments of longtime, older residents:

> "I used to know people; now I see many strangers."
>
> "They take over everything. . . ."
>
> "Because we've got an accent, they think we're slow."

"They" were "incomers," many of them working in the cities and living in the country.

Dimensions of Deprivation

The aging locals felt their ties fragmenting, not only as the youth left, but also as their traditional pride-of-workplace eroded. Conglomerates had bought up small family-run mines and quarries. Mechanization had reduced the quarry workforce by between 50 percent and 75 percent in 20 years. Firms increasingly used contract labor, reducing not only the number of jobs, but also the networks among the workers who remained.

The social gap between the old and the newcomers seemed too wide for recreating the community "glue" that the locals sensed was disappearing. People spoke of the village "losing its roots." Incomers were "nice people" but with "town ways." "The only time I see them," one longtime resident said, "is when they're snowed in and need help."

The other major source of income, as well as stability and security, was farming. Small farms were being bought up by "business people" and "hobby farmers," or otherwise made economically vulnerable by the large reduction in subsidies under the new agricultural policies of the European Union. Since the area was one of acknowledged natural beauty, conveniently off the main road, it attracted many tourists and the services of the tourist industry, as well as the low-wage jobs that are typical in the tourist trade.

While perhaps a majority of local people regarded themselves as economically better-off than a decade before—many tenants of public housing, for example, had taken advantage of the 1986 right-to-buy legislation—they were also acutely aware of the fragility of their bounty. At least a third of the households in some villages had weekly incomes much lower than the national average. Yet many people were simply unaware of the availability of welfare information and income support services. They had poor access to health centers, supermarkets, job centers, and social welfare services, although most felt they had a neighbor they could turn to for advice.

Other signs of an information gap were the large majority who were unsure about who made important political decisions for their area. At the same time there was a diffuse sense of antagonism toward the Hill Park Planning Board, the national entity charged with conserving and enhancing the district.

These changes evoked a sense among the locals, perhaps shared by those in similar areas in Europe and North America, of a future in which newcomers replaced the old ways with a set of urban values for assessing the worth of others: mainly signs of affluence like occupational status, house, car, and consumer durables. In this new order, many low-paid villagers would be assigned a place close to the bottom on the social ladder, the study on deprivation reported in 1991.

National Hill Park Board

Regardless of the feelings the Hill Park District's older residents had about the National Hill Park Planning Board, they had an empathetic advocate sitting on the board who believed in the board's mission and was impatient with its limitations. It could not carry out what it planned. The official duties of the board were to protect and enhance the natural beauty, provide for public enjoyment, and take account of the social and economic well-being of those who lived and worked in the area.

As a result of apparent organizational gridlock, the board's most active member and district advocate concluded there should be a closer relationship between planning and service delivery, especially in relation to housing and economic development. This was a view later reinforced by the commissioned report for the new Hill Park Trust. The trust was set up at the board's initiative through a wealthy businessman who agreed to incorporate it as a nonprofit foundation in 1987. Its mission was to preserve and develop both the natural heritage of the area and address the problems of counterurbanization faced by the locals. Appealing to both the social and material values in philanthropy and business, the trust produced an endowment of almost $4 million within three years.

Parent to Innovation

The trust, under a strategically selected board of donors, experts in fiscal and legal matters, and regional public decision makers, hired a small staff in mid-1988. With operating costs of about $55,000, supported by small grants from the Countryside Commission, other trusts and local village councils, and business firms, the trust immediately undertook small projects in collaboration with local groups. It initiated a low-cost housing development of 20 units with a number of local churches and voluntary societies, funded environmental conservation projects, historic building preservation, and education and social welfare programs.

Sources of an Idea

Well before commissioning the report on the district, the Hill Park board's chair and advisor to the trust learned of an innovation in community economic development through his European ties. As head of the European Council for Villages and Small Towns (ECOVAST), he supported the view that telecommunications could offset rural disadvantages of remoteness and sparse populations. He learned about the "community teleservice center" or "electronic village hall" developing in Scandinavia. It had been inspired by none other than the United Kingdom's Open University, the countrywide unique off-campus, degree-awarding education system. The teleservice concept proffered a social milieu for use of telecommunications and a bridge for those who were unfamiliar with the new information technologies (Watkins 1990).

The Swedish Model

Although the idea, also known as the "telecottage," was born in Denmark, it was first set up in Vemdalen, a remote village in northern Sweden, in 1985. Employment there from forestry and tourism was in decline, and the population was shrinking as the younger generation went to work in the cities of the south. Swedish authorities and the public telephone carrier provided the $200,000 in funds for these electronic centers that brought computers and telecommunications to rural villages, some of which had no such technology. They were in tune with Swedish government efforts to maintain viable rural communities by moving industry into the countryside to prevent outmigration. The telecottages performed distance work for governmental units and other organizations, and included tasks such as scanning precomputer-era paper files into computerized records and returning them by telephone lines or satellite to the contractor (including the military bureaucracy). About four in ten villagers used the telecottage; over half the work was skilled and well paid (Denbigh 1991).

The Nordic Association of Telecottages, with about 50 member sites in the early 1990s, began in Vemdalen and expanded into Telecottages International to spread the experience of running telecottages around the world. There had been initial doubts about the telecottages in the mid-1980s by Swedish labor unions who saw a kind of old-time, home-based, piece-rate worker; typically "some poor girl in the northern part of Sweden being exploited by a big company in southern Sweden"—low paid, not having a vacation or other entitlements, required to cook for her family, and at the same time having to sit at the computer screen. Following a three-year study, the unions found that the typical teleworker was a man between 30 and 40 years old, one so valuable to his company that it did not say "no" when he asked to work at home. The union then began to establish telecottages for its own members, who, as home-based teleworkers, used the union for social contact and solidarity. They went in at least once a week to discuss their work plans (Albrechtsen 1991). This system effectively dealt with two of the main issues of distance work: social isolation on the part of the employee, and managerial supervision (BT 1989; ORA 1992).

Fertile Ground

This picture of a telematics innovation, another version of community information technology, was enthusiastically reported back to the Hill Park Trust and to other potential U.K. adopters, such as Action with Rural Communities in England (ACRE), a network of rural community councils (Denbigh 1991). ACRE's mission, according to its president, was to "work to sustain living village communities." It began to see the telecottage as "a new weapon in the armory of rural development . . . not a panacea for all ills, but it can certainly offer a solution to many problems." ACRE used its resources to "communicate and catalyze the idea" through the mass media and put interested people in touch with each other. Through its own network, it informed them of funding and assistance.

Strongly spurred by the Hill Park Trust, ACRE brought together its leading members and decided to seek funds for a staff consultant on teleworking at the end of the 1980s. The position was funded by British Telecom (BT), the giant telecommunications carrier, and became a nucleus around which incipient interest could solidify.

The Technology Landscape

The telecottage message readily took hold in the Hill Park Trust and in dozens of other places in the United Kingdom. In several respects, the ground had been laid early in the 1980s by the British government. Spurred in the mid-seventies by the commercial success of American computer games, British home computer producers were able to increase their market fivefold by 1985, outstripping the United States, and creating a computer-conscious public (Haddon and Skinner 1991).

The government promoted the market by a campaign—"There is no future without IT"—and encouraged computer awareness and literacy through policy incentives and programs. The Department of Industry provided funds intended to make England the first country to have a computer in every classroom. It also began an IT support program for people with special needs, supporting firms that would use IT to offer goods and services to people with disabilities who worked in services such as education, rehabilitation, and remote worksites. It sponsored in-home IT training projects to improve employable skills, and set up accreditation and certification standards for trainers and trainees (Department of Trade and Industry 1992).

These activities also encouraged the formation of IT consultancies for both industry and government to support development of training programs, materials, and computerware for special groups (IT World 1992a). By the late eighties, city governments in partnership with public and private donors and experts offered in-home training for mentally and physically disabled people and their caregivers, and women with child care responsibilities. Trainees were loaned all necessary computer equipment for the duration of the courses. These were self-paced and supported by a hotline and home visits by a trainer (IT World 1992b).

The British Broadcasting Corporation promoted the computer culture by offering programs on IT with hands-on options. In addition, the Open University, renowned as an accessible source for adult education, carried out degree-granting programs in its study centers and by home-based learning throughout the country. It was ahead of many adult learning institutions in the early 1970s, when it installed computer terminals in 200 of its centers. With the upsurge of computing in the eighties, the university extended its computer access beyond the school and university centers into libraries, and later developed a home computing policy. This allowed students to take computer courses, and obtain equipment and materials at discounted prices through pooled purchasing with central government grants. By the early nineties, the courses and number of students had quadrupled (Qvortrup 1992).

From Idea to Tactics

In spite of a rich awareness of telematics possibilities and a generally enabling social climate, the Hill Park Trust's new staff director knew virtually nothing in practical terms about computers. He had a background in urban community development, a kind of soft technology in the form of on-the-ground grass roots organizing. Unable to visualize the idea of a telecottage, he mentally filed away the concept with a footnote, "What the hell are these things, a franchise package?"

As fiscal pressures and the need for the trust to present an enticing and effective area development strategy loomed ever larger, a British telecottage appeared to be a plausible option—if it could be something more substantial than a vague description, and if it could be made usable within the constraining realities of the United Kingdom and the Hill

Park District. The trust learned from the now privatized British Telecom about its tax-exempt Community Fund, which sought to develop rural projects and included using restored historic buildings as telecottages.

Nexus of Private and Public Interests

British Telecom had recently agreed to finance, with Scottish economic development authorities, an extensive, state-of-the-art telecommunications infrastructure. It would provide an all-digital system for the rural areas of Scotland, including more than 90 sparsely populated islands, amounting to over $20 million (Watt 1991). The Scots needed new industry and new jobs; BT would clearly benefit by expanding its market. Home-based BT teleworkers from Scotland would provide telephone directory assistance (HIDB 1989). Its operators would have video-voice contact with their supervisors and colleagues. BT expected to have 2 million such workers by the mid-1990s.

BT's market research forecast 4 to 5 million teleworkers in the United Kingdom by mid-decade, saving 20 percent of commuting miles, with 185 fewer traffic deaths and 11,000 fewer injuries at a net annual gain to the economy of $185 million from savings in health care, policing, and car fuel. Projections also showed higher housing prices in some areas and lower ones in others. The most serious effect would occur in food service and mass transit jobs. But overall, these losses would be offset by job increases in residential areas (Watkins 1990).

After BT settled its contract in the Highlands, it looked for other options for telecommunications site development, such as teleservice centers, according to a BT managerial officer. This was the impetus for its offer to the Hill Park Trust.

Decision to Adopt

At this point the trust's top priority was to find a way to capture development resources; it was more than willing to be courted. It proposed a joint site visit to Sweden, supported by BT, to learn about the electronic centers. The Swedish visit confirmed the value of the telecottage concept: a supportable and potentially effective community development strategy for the trust, and as indicated in a BT marketing management report, "an excellent way of exploiting the benefits of modern telecommunications and information technology. . . . An important opportunity for BT to be seen as supporting an innovative and radical solution to the growing problems in rural areas."

The U.K. visitors noted that many Swedish teleservice centers focused on services to disadvantaged groups, such as the blind and disabled, which were not readily feasible in the United Kingdom. The United Kingdom lacked comparable political and public support and resources to finance such services.

However, the more business-oriented focus adopted by some of the centers could work in the United Kingdom. Therefore, BT concluded that it should support and encourage teleservice centers. This would address some of the major problems of telecommunications in rural areas, generate BT equipment and network sales, and perhaps bring public relations gains from community action in the localities. The Swedish telecommunications monopoly had seen sales growth through its use of the centers as display and demonstration sites. Small businesses often purchased their own equipment once they realized that they needed dedicated apparatus (BT 1989).

Shortly after its joint visit to Sweden, while the trust laid its IT plans, BT contributed substantial funds to another—the first—English telecottage located in northeast Britain. It opened at the end of 1989. This step gave BT an immediate gain of favorable publicity. Its grants of start-up funds and equipment were noted as one of the few sources for telecottage development. As interpreted for the public by the British press:

> If the telecottage idea being tried out in rural communities were to be adopted nationwide, the problem of unemployment, lack of affordable training and long-term shortage of information technology skills could well be solved.
>
> A telecottage is a workplace-cum-training center in the heart of a village. It provides the local community with low cost access to information technology they could not otherwise afford. . . . The telecottage can be an electronic sorting office, mailbox and notice board, and electronic reference library, a word and data processing service bureau, a desktop publishing house, a teleshop, and a support center for teleworkers and local businesses. (Harnett 1991)

The Hill Park Telebusiness Center

The Hill Park Trust and BT began their venture the next year. The partners had at least some converging interests in community IT. But in the words of the trust's director, telecottages were "just rooms with computers . . . nothing special; . . . it's what you do with them—their goals and organization—that makes them new and different." And the trust wanted its telecottage to be special.

The trust conceived its telebusiness center as an infrastructure for business development, the only one to be organized as a private management, profit-making venture in the United Kingdom, following its goal to create a sustainable, supportive economic development tool for the region.

It subcontracted the management of the center to a small firm that offered consultant and training services in personnel and facilities management. The new management advertised the telebusiness center as a "new preview center" where clients could now view multimedia products and courseware in picturesque Hill Park and have access to a wide range of high-technology information services and equipment.

The property itself, including the now renovated farm buildings costing over a half-million dollars, was estimated to be worth $1.2 million. The trust could arrange a generous management contract that would last until 1998 because it held a 99-year property lease at a "peppercorn rent" from the landowner quarry firm. The contract provided a year's free rent. The center's IT and telecommunications equipment, worth $20,000, was donated by BT. The center also housed a main office, including coffee lounge and conference room.

The trust received rent from tenants in the 11 available office suites. A package of basic services, to be provided by and reimbursed to the management firm, were included in the office rental fee. Included in the basic services package were reception, messaging, secretarial services, free business consultation one day per month, basic utilities and maintenance, use of equipment, and conference and coffee facilities. The firm would also obtain earnings by providing additional services such as training programs, consultation, and information media production and sales. Thus both the management firm and the trust had a mutual interest in making the center self-sustaining. The firm estimated that it would need at least five or six steady tenants in order to break even.

Early Users

The first four tenants were small local businesses of a wide variety. The first, a computer graphics firm, soon left to relocate in a large, urban-based advertising company. Another, a local couple, conducted training programs to help local women learn about public health regulations for beginning child care centers. The other two tenants were a local woman management consultant and the U.K. headquarters of an Australian software firm.

Services

Other services that the center offered as a provider or on a self-serve basis for tenants and others ranged from bookkeeping and mailing to desktop publishing, fax, copying, conferencing, and translation services. With the growing presence of the European Union, the languages of business were becoming diverse. Helped by the local Rural Development

Commission, the Hill Park Telebusiness Center had a listing of translator subcontractors who were fluent in European languages as well as Russian and Japanese.

In addition to the business training that its management firm would provide, the center contracted with local training and enterprise councils to offer additional courses funded by government vocational education monies. In time, the center hoped to have a program in IT and self-marketing skills that would entitle participants to both U.K. and European Union–wide skills certification.

Other center objectives, such as encouraging voluntary groups to use center services, establishing ties with the education authority, and linking with home-based individuals and corporations for telework and telelearning, were not pursued in the early years due to business-focused priorities and limited staff. The trust viewed its "market" as 200 local businesses, a number of large urban areas from greater Manchester to Leeds and Sheffield in northcentral England, and the entire country and even the world, given the center's telecommunications capability.

Prelude to Phase II

In less than 18 months, the center reached its initial goals of providing high-technology workspace facilities and services in a historically preserved site under entrepreneurial management. Its business objectives were under way. Its broader community focus, to educate and support local groups for voluntary action, had not really begun and remained for the trust to initiate. Recruiting distance work first meant having a qualified local tele-workforce that could work at the center or at home. This could mean better-paid work in the Hill Park country, and the possibility of young families being able to afford housing in the area. A significant step toward this goal had been made by obtaining donations of classroom furnishings and ten computers from the post office and BT by mid-1992.

Basis for the Partnership Mosaic

The trust foresaw a fiscal balance if the center's in-kind resource suppliers and a mosaic of others could be retained as partners. The more than $600,000 needed for the special historic and high-technology renovation and development of the site (most centers required a minimum of $25,000 to $30,000) was negotiated with many organizations by the trust, each of whom had a stake in the promise of the center.

BT's marketing interest was clear. The center was the first to which it gave cash, almost $100,000, perhaps because it was the first to have a profit-making focus. With funds coming from its tax-free foundation, it could be seen as supportive of rural heritage preservation at the same time that it developed its telecommunications market.

The major contributor to the project, however, was the Rural Development Commission (RDC) whose task was to develop workspaces, usually interpreted as office building construction. The trust was able to convince the RDC that creating workspaces in the telecottage was more suitable to the culture and environment of the region than an office complex. RDC then agreed to put up half the total start-up costs at about $300,000. But the bargain was a hard one. It wanted half of the center's income for the next 20 years, a demand that the trust would attempt to renegotiate.

In addition to a few thousand dollars from small local government councils that wanted to promote employment in environmentally sensitive ways, two other significant grantors became involved when the trust managed to play the interests of one against the other. Two large local government councils, one led by the Labor Party, the other by the conservative Tories, matched each other with two $40,000 grants for the telecottage. The Labor-led council (whose political position was similar to the trust's staff's) was not initially interested because its constituency was mainly urban workers. It agreed to become a funder after the Tory-led council provided funds; Labor could not be seen to be outdone in such a community-supporting act by the conservatives. The monies from the Tory council, by coincidence, came about when its council chair noticed that he and a prestigious trust board member had gone to an elite school together decades ago and sought a means to renew and develop that useful tie.

A second major set of supporters were several training and enterprise councils (TECs) responsible for providing job training programs. Their local activity had been hampered by a lack of workspace in which fledgling firms could develop. One TEC, which had been using a mobile unit, was assisting the center in developing training programs and would use the center as a site for its own efforts. Another newly forming TEC, seeking to demonstrate its commitment to rural areas in order to qualify for a TEC government grant, contributed almost $40,000.

Another partner that stood to gain from the success of the center was the National Hill Park Planning Board, from which the trust and telecottage were born. It provided over $25,000 to assist in the preservation of the site, following its mandate.

The center's free use (at a "peppercorn rent") of land granted by the quarrying firm landowner assured the firm of careful, no cost management, preservation, and improvement of very valuable property.

The agreement also relieved it of any future environmental regulatory expenses and enhanced its public image at a time when, by reducing its local workforce, it was not very popular.

The funds, equipment, facilities, services, and expertise from all the collaborators, melded in a timely way by the trust, were necessary to the creation of the center. At the same time, each was expecting their contribution to bring them a return on their investment within the foreseeable future and over the longer term.

Prospects

The immediate fiscal outlook for the center was good. It had no outstanding debt, and its operating costs could be met by the current renters of three to four workspaces. Should its management firm not be able to make a profit or break even over the contract period of six years, the trust had several options. It could provide free rent to the firm or allow it to retain some of the tenant rental fees; it could hire another firm on a profit-sharing basis. It could also become a TEC center by applying for central government funds to offer certifiable vocational and adult skills training to strengthen worker employability and business success.

Weaving a New Net

The center could afford to be patient because of its cushion of valuable real estate. But most telecottages were only poorly endowed. For them to have a secure start-up period would, in the view of the trust, require a five-year grant to cover annual operating expenses of about $25,000 and a full-time program manager at about $30,000, in addition to initial renovation and technology costs. Others have made lower estimates and managed on somewhat fewer resources (Denbigh 1991).

Even in its early stage of development, the trust's staff, aware of the paucity of staff resources, and the necessity of getting the innovative message of the center to the local community and general public, got the support of ACRE for another joint step. They persuaded BT to expand the work of the ACRE telecottage consultant through a separate new organization. It would promote telecottages and coordinate the joint activities of the now 40 to 50 telecottages that were developing across England and Wales. With a three-year grant of $140,000 from BT, the Telecottage Association was launched in 1993, supported also by the Rural Development Commission and other donors.

The Telecottage Association

The association's mission was "to improve the condition of people in greatest need, particularly in rural areas, by seeking to develop local economies through the use of shared information technology and telecommunications facilities based at telecottages. Telecottages provide an access point to training in new skills, access to employment, and access to information."

It explicitly sought, based on the focus of the majority of its members, not to be seen as a purely commercial group of enterprisers, but wanted to "promote the community benefits of telecottages—this is what sets them apart from purely commercial enterprises . . . promote the use of telecottages to potential users, including people with special needs." It also wanted to "establish links with, and a database on, agencies who can offer assistance . . . with national leaders (e.g., members of Parliament) who can further these objectives . . . and national and international links with organizations with similar objectives . . ." (Business Plan 1992). Finally, it was to act as a public relations and media organization for telecottages, using key spokespeople within the movement to help telecottages achieve balance between commercial and community objectives, and represent their views in European IT discussions.

Diverse Sister Centers

The program of the telecottages came to be a balance between community development—nurturing local groups, schools, churches, and the disadvantaged—and economic development, supporting local businesses and bringing in work and jobs. The different paths taken depended on the priorities of the funding sources. Since most of the money and facilities accessible locally were from local government councils and organizations, many new telecottages had a community development focus, at least initially.

Shaping the Center at Fielding for Social Needs

Just as the sources of funds and other resources helped shape the program and priorities of the Hill Park Telebusiness Center, the same idea planted in a different situation produced a very different kind of telecottage. Fielding was another rural agricultural and quarrying area, with only about 2,800 people living in several tiny villages covering four miles. Its telecottage took a community development path to economic improvement rather than itself becoming a profit-making, business support enterprise.

At about the time that the trust raised the telecottage issue in Hill Park in the late eighties, it also presented the idea to the town council of Fielding, another town facing the same daunting task of economic development. The council had the local school authority develop a telecottage within its Community Education Project, a job training program.

The telecottage was located at the local school and was funded by the Rural Development Commission, the county council, and several educational institutions. It received IT hardware from BT during its foray into telecottages. Initially, costs were saved by having school staff supervise the activities.

The program offered services to local voluntary groups and small businesses. These ranged from certifiable vocational training for youth and adults to IT support and training, community resource information access, and use for formal classroom instruction. According to the program's director, its tenor was meant to be "small and accessible and user-friendly. . . . The informal aspects of the telecottage, its coffee bar, and drop-in center, along with other activities for allowing people to stay in touch with people and for networking, ought not be underestimated." In response to this atmosphere an author wrote that it was "an oasis in a writer's desert." A local candidate designed her own campaign flyer with the center's IT:

> Liberal democrats: Annie Taylor, the best choice for our new county councilor. Annie Taylor is for: school for the rising fives; pupils and students with special needs; more support for playgroups; more home helps and expansion of the Meals on Wheels service; more police on our streets; a cleaner, greener environment. Annie Taylor is against: the abolition of school meals; cuts in the funding of Somerset's colleges; the sale of county farms; the county council's failure to support the school re-building programme; the county's failure to support the new library.

In addition, the local pub produced its menus on the telecottage computer. The local "Health Visitor" also helped women in the community by setting up a telecottage course designed to take the mystique out of computers; 30 people came on the first evening after one advertisement in the local paper.

Managing the Future

The purposes of the primary goals of the funders at Fielding were clearly educational and were to serve the public interest using public resources. While it also planned to become a teleworking center, a site for home-based computer workers to do their jobs, "we found this to be a lot more difficult. Many home workers have left the community behind and are not likely to use telecottages on a regular basis unless they are really nearby and easily reached. . . . We originally planned that within three years the telecottage would be economically self-supporting. . . . It will take a bit longer. . . . We're in no hurry."

To widen the scope of services and take advantage of new sources of funds, the Fielding telecottage won a grant from the European Union's Social Fund, targeted to rural areas:

> Half the European population still lives outside major conurbations. . . . Quality of life and employment opportunities in the rural areas of Europe are under threat. . . . Rural areas will need information technology, telecommunications and broadcasting infrastructures comparable to urban centers if they are to develop a more balanced economic activity with diversity of employment. . . . Telematic systems linked to better telecommunications can facilitate economic growth in rural areas by allowing new forms of employment to be located in rural communities. Jobs can be moved to people. . . . (ORA 1992)

Other ways to promote user interest in the telecottage were successfully pursued by sister telecottages. Several telecottages led their villages in undertaking a Village Appraisal, a computer software program promoted across the country by ACRE. Aimed at town organizations and residents, it assisted survey development, including suggested questions, data compilation, analysis, and reporting, as well as guidance on community input in the development and conduct of the survey itself (Bellamy 1991). The aim was to learn from and inform residents, public bodies, and businesses about the priority issues of the community, and to encourage discussion about how to address unemployment and education issues, and about the place of IT in finding solutions. In the process, people learned about the services of the telecottage.

Another telecottage thrust was to become an information access point by accessing databases of community interest, both on-line and by satellite. These included employer job offerings throughout the country; planning and construction regulations and procedures; entitlement programs and application processes; satellite weather and TV programs, and tourist travel and accommodation listings. Some telecottages become Open University access points, connecting adults to courses and degree-granting institutions across the country.

Summary: Environment, Enigmas, Answers

The institution that was to oversee the environment and well-being of the Hill Park countryside, the National Hill Park Planning Board, saw that it could not carry out its mission in the climate of the 1980s. Threatening conditions included outmigration of jobs and young families and immigration of urban professionals among disillusioned, aged locals in economic decline; inaccessible housing and services; and new laws that weakened the county councils that once addressed the problems. To give itself an instrument for action, the board used its resource-rich social network to create an endowed trust to allow it to grant funds to local groups to deal with some of the social needs.

These efforts were only to establish its good intentions before the public, a prelude to a wider vision: an economic development strategy for the area, showcased as the Hill Park Telebusiness Center, a telecottage. Inspired by the United Kingdom's Open University, and originally conceived in Denmark, implemented in Sweden, and reported in the European Union, the telecottage concept returned to the United Kingdom in many variants. The conduits to the United Kingdom were the trust's European links and its U.K. network, Action with Rural Communities in England. To anchor and promote interest in the telecottage as both an adaptable concept and a usable, somewhat tested model for community development, the trust obtained staff support through funds from the newly privatized and high-profit British Telecom.

The ground was fertile for using information technology to support community economic and social development throughout the British countryside, whose straits were similar to the Hill Park District. The central government promoted IT to advance the economy, and initiated projects in industry, job training, and IT support centers. The public information and education media, BBC and the Open University, alerted and enabled the public to use IT.

But more important than a supportive environment was BT's offer of resources for its own purposes of setting up sites to expand its IT market, preparing isolated sites for its distance worker (teleworker) plans, and being seen as community-friendly. These interests meshed with the trust's need to produce a visible, cutting edge development program. After the on-site visit to Sweden that allowed both BT and the trust to envision a U.K.–style telecottage, BT's first cash grant for a center confirmed the joint undertaking. Drawing in other potential stakeholders, local town councils, the Rural Development Commission, and job training programs, the trust merged sufficient funds, equipment, facilities, services, and expertise to begin the Hill Park Telebusiness Center. It had convinced each participant that the prospective gains for its own organizational purposes would be worth the costs.

Recognizing that interest in the telecottage idea was outstripping the resources to manage it, the trust staff led the growing network of centers in persuading BT to fund the start-up of an information and promotion Telecottage Association. This group supported the telecottages and nurtured interest in them. It provided local groups with the experience of seasoned centers, sources of funds, and expert contacts that were essential to development of any variant of telecenter—economic, educational, or social. Such support could save not only time and start-up costs, but could also prevent some of the frustration and discouragement that led to unknown numbers of aborted telecenters.

References

Albrechtsen, H. 1991. "Lessons from Abroad." In *Telecottages Today*, edited by A. Denbigh. Gloucester, United Kingdon: Action with Rural Communities in England (ACRE).

Bellamy, D. 1991. *Community Computers in Connection with the Welsh Local Jigsaw Campaign*. Cardiff, Wales: Natural Economy Research Unit, National Museum of Wales.

British Telecom (BT). 1989. *Swedish Telecottages: Telecommunications in Rural Areas*. Internal Report. London: British Telecom, Marketing Operations and Planning, October.

Business Plan. 1992. *The Telecottage Association*. Gloucestershire, United Kingdom.

Denbigh, A., ed. 1991. *Telecottages Today*. Gloucestershire, United Kingdom: Action with Rural Communities in England (ACRE), August.

Department of Trade and Industry. 1992. *Home Delivered Training. Information Technology Vocational Skills*. London: DTI, HM Government.

Haddon, L., and D. Skinner. 1991. "The Enigma of the Micro: Lessons from the British Home Computer Boom." *Social Science Computer Review* 9 (3): 435–50.

Harnett, J. 1991. *Microvillage Industry*. The Guardian (UK), 30 May.

Highlands and Islands Development Board (HIDB). 1989. *New Initiative to Put Highlands and Islands at Forefront of Communications Technology*. Top Business (UK), November.

IT World. 1992a. *Competencies in Technology Transfer, Teleworking, and Teletraining*. London: IT World Consultants.

———. 1992b. *Computer Skills Training at Home in East Birmingham*. Interim Report. London: IT World.

Office of Rural Assistance (ORA). 1992. *Research and Technology on Telematics in Rural Areas*. Brussels, Belgium: European Commission.

Qvortrup, L. 1992. *Learning at a Distance*. Zurich, Switzerland: Center for Teleservice Centers International.

Watkins, C., ed. 1990. *Teleworking and Telecottages*. Gloucestershire, UK: Centre for Rural Studies, Royal Agricultural College.

Watt, J. 1991. *Community Teleservice Centres in the Highlands and Islands of Scotland: A Progress Report*. Edinburgh, Scotland: Highlands and Islands Development Board.

SECTION D
Responsive Government

Community empowerment, taking place concurrently and catalyzed by the newly emerging hybrid professional, results from community involvement, community participation, and community organization around issues of health and quality of life.

Helen Grace, *Building Community*, Kellogg Foundation, 1990

CHAPTER

12

INFORMATION TECHNOLOGY AND PARTICIPATORY DEMOCRACY

THE PROMISE of the new information technologies is in their potential to extend the powers of people's talents, replace drudgery with convenience at work and home, and foster new forms of social relations and education. A still larger possibility is one that goes beyond the capacity and day-to-day concerns of single individuals.

Across the more than two centuries of U.S. history, changes in information technology have enabled wider participation in the public decision making that affects personal and community life, the choices that build the health-supporting infrastructure in its largest sense. The how and the what of political life—timely and usable information about current issues and how to affect them—has reached larger and more diverse audiences, from town crier to the penny press, telegraph, telephone, and radio and television (Ladd 1989). As a result, the gatekeepers of political communication have shifted from local newspaper owners to legislative representatives, party leaders, and TV news analysts (OTA 1990). The burgeoning and converging of the new information technologies may change political life even more than in the past, and perhaps far faster.

The Uncertain State of Public Participation

In the suburban enclaves and affluent cities and towns of California, the users of networked computers join in electronic discussions from their homes. Only about one in five users communicate from public terminals in libraries and other public sites (Furger 1992). By one estimate, home computer users mainly do word processing; about a third engage in communications (which requires a modem-telephone link), and a similar number use educational programs (OTA 1990). In the older, more industrial cities of the Midwest, the vision of "teledemocracy" was the inspiration for the development of citywide "freenets" in the 1980s.

Citizens suddenly had at their fingertips current information about activities at all levels of government: agendas, decisions, and decision makers; candidates, their backgrounds, and their views (NPTN 1993). On some networks, however, political comments form only about 5 percent of the messages (OTA 1990). In other recent surveys, between 35 and 60 percent of Americans said they were interested in policy issues such as health, the economy, the environment, and new technologies (Office of Disease Prevention 1994). But the depth of this interest and the opportunity and incentives to participate in policy processes at any level of public life vary widely.

Whatever democratic fruits electronic nets hold, those who have gained most so far are those who already have the most, people whose incomes are about double the national average. Those with the best access to the information media, especially through computer-based systems, are higher-income, better-educated people, while those with least access to public affairs information are people with low incomes. Other sources of information and communication, not surprisingly, are also linked to higher income and education: newspapers, books, library use, cable, videotex, and VCRs (OTA 1990).

Universal access is based on the free or guaranteed access to broadcast TV and telephone services. Even here, the 6 million homes that have no telephone are mainly headed by single, poor women with small children. Others are people who live in public housing or hotels (Benton Foundation).

As far as can be determined, the overwhelming use of home-based technologies is for personal interactions and support, advice rendering, and entertainment. For example, in the mid-1980s, almost half of computer buyers thought they would use their machines for education, but only about one in ten actually did so (Roth 1987).

Other conduits of civic information and action, such as school, church, business, labor, health, and environmental groups, involve few Americans beyond basic attendance at open meetings. From 2 percent to 7 percent of adults in the United States are part of decision-making units in such groups, although about 9 percent of African American adults belong to church boards. Government-related bodies garner the least participation (1.5 percent or less), and greater participation in organizational decision-making bodies comes from people with more than a high school education (Groups and Associations 1988).

At the end of the twentieth century, even minimal political participation in the form of political awareness, knowledge, and voting is on the decline, and it seems that well-educated and affluent Americans are the citizens who feel they have a stake in what happens and can make a difference (Ornstein et al. 1988). At the same time, the demands for governmental and interstate action have increased worldwide on issues ranging from security and trade to environment and communications. (Transnational corporations are now large enough to challenge the power of some governments.) All of this is further complicated by the ambivalence of Americans about how much government should do. On one hand, they want limited government, believing it is wasteful and too controlling over daily life. On the other, they want it to help people meet health and education needs as well as help those who are poor (Ladd 1989).

Potential for New Political Forms

As the new technologies become a growing part of this political mix, the imperatives of governance and of political access will change for good or ill, depending on the policies that are now being framed and the patterns that flow from them. IT has become essential for effective and efficient government, for legitimate national security, law enforcement, revenue collection, financial transactions, and program administration. But these benefits have their counterparts in potential abuse, such as political surveillance and intrusions on personal, financial, health, and social privacy. Such abuses can be prevented only if policies and systems are designed to prevent them (OTA 1990).

New guarantees of political access that are appropriate to the new IT environment can help ensure that the policy changes that are shaping the information infrastructure will be adequate to controlling abuses and enabling effective public participation. Although in principal everyone might be able to discuss public issues with officials and others, they will not be able to do so in practice without access to the hardware, software, skills, and navigational tools to find and use the benefits of the electronic world and to use the new tools in ways as accessible as the penny press, universal phone service, and the broadcast media of previous decades.

Those who have access could become their own gatekeepers and publishers of information. But such options depend on who the system gatekeepers are: the owners of networks and information sources, the rulemakers and regulators, the independent watchdogs. Apart from letter writing and visits to officials, demonstrations, or running for office, most participation is indirect—most commonly through voting. Even active citizens have their voice heard through some chosen group, whether a political party, occupational group, profession, union, or interest group involved in business, church, civil rights, environmental, or health and social welfare issues. These groups voice members' concerns and preferences, recruit policymakers to their cause, and persuade the public and voters. Throughout all these activities, they collect, develop, and disseminate information. None of these policy-relevant actions could be sustained by individuals acting alone.

The new technologies are changing the conduct and effectiveness of political campaigns, allowing, for example, analysis and coverage of party campaigns and opinion polls, as well as immediate responses to others' actions and views. The other side of the coin is that IT enables candidates to manipulate citizens' perceptions of issues and personalities, and allows them to be less accountable to political parties by relying more on political consultants. Alternatively, the new technologies could revive the role of parties by creating voter databases and other resources to be made available to candidates, not on the basis of ability to pay but on the commitment to the party's perspective on the issues (OTA 1990).

Public Interest Groups

Using the resources of the Internet, some public interest groups have moved several steps beyond individual citizen awareness and voter literacy campaigns to organized political action. They conduct ongoing dialogs with other groups and elected and other officials. They identify like-minded people, create new interest groups, raise financial and political support, and track government activities. Using computer-based public data, they analyze, graphically present, publicize, and press for legislative and policy changes on issues from national policy action to local environmental protection and arson control (Taxpayer 1993; OTA 1990).

Policy Activity

In the late 1970s, the U.S. Department of Justice compiled the world's largest on-line national government legal database. The system, called JURIS, contains extensive information on federal case law from the U.S. Supreme Court and federal court system, public laws from Congress, regulations, executive orders, attorney general opinions, and administrative law on government ethics, equal employment, labor law, and environmental protection.

In the 1980s, the Justice Department contracted a private firm to supply the database to the public on a commercial basis, costing users $4 to $6 per minute through a commercial computer network. When the contract was being renegotiated in 1993, a public interest group, the Taxpayer Assets Project (TAP), led a drive to provide free public access to it. Through the Internet, it notified several hundred lawyers, computer professionals, librarians, public interest groups, and others across the country. TAP also contacted the U.S. Attorney General and selected members of Congress, and wrote editorials and articles in relevant media. As a result of the e-mail messages, several hundred network users wrote the Justice Department and their own congressional representatives. The result was the granting of public access to JURIS and the withdrawal of the private firm's contract bid (Taxpayer 1993). Although communication of timely information through the Internet was not the sole ingredient of this successful public interest activity, it made possible the timely, coordinated, and focused response that would otherwise have been much more expensive, unwieldy, and perhaps not as inclusive or effective.

Environmental Action

The Environmental Protection Agency (EPA), under the Community Right to Know Act of the late 1980s, made available to the public its Toxic Release Inventory (TRI) on toxic chemical emissions by thousands of facilities. The formats included paper reports, computer diskettes, electronic databases, and CD-ROM disks. A survey of user groups, about 150 respondents of the more than 200 state, citizen, and industry groups sampled, showed that this information spurred joint citizen-industry action at the local level, most often among the citizen groups. It also stimulated lobbying for stronger legislative, regulatory, and administrative action. The formats preferred by the 47 state and 67 citizen and environmental groups were the hard copies and diskettes, while the 19 industry groups preferred the EPA technical databases, each type of group preferring the format that best suited its technological capacity (Lynn and Koebrick 1992).

Most importantly, the survey found that individual citizens most often turned first to citizen groups to learn about and effectively use the TRI (GAO 1991). The legal availability of the information was not sufficient to bring about environmental improvements. The groups became a bridge, a conduit, a necessary intermediary for community action (Lynn et al. 1992). They also served as interpreters of the databases to the press. Fewer than one in five reporters used the EPA data directly; most of them based their stories on the reports of citizen organizations that accessed the data (MacLean and Orum 1992).

The right to know is then not the same as an effective right to act. Effective action to influence public opinion and regulatory rule making, to seek legal redress or engage in direct negotiation, requires additional tools besides data. Such tools include organizational support, technical expertise, legal assistance, and more and better access to information in more user-friendly formats (Settina and Orum 1991). In every instance where local citizen action was effective, the EPA information was only one ingredient, albeit an important one, among several ingredients, including previous organized advocacy, public opinion formation, getting press coverage, petition and letter-writing campaigns, and coalition-building. The addition of credible evidence in accessible, graphic forms then was a spur to further, more effective progress toward local goals of reducing exposure to chemical hazards.

Since the survey report, EPA information and communication have been enhanced by the federally sponsored right to know electronic network (RTKnet) developed through the action of public interest groups.

Housing Advocacy

While it is difficult for any individual to learn about and make effective use of public information for community purposes, the problems are multiplied for those whose live in disadvantaged communities. This reality makes community-based bridging organizations even more important. In one low-income neighborhood in Brooklyn, New York, a community development organization focused on rehabilitation and management of city-owned apartment buildings, tenant organizing and training for cooperative management, and commercial development. It complemented its program with a computerized Arson Risk Prediction Index (Cook 1985). The index could predict a third of potential arsons and analyze eight sources of public data. It then reported profiles and patterns among buildings and owners.

The strengths and limits of the index, however, did not lie in such factual information. The organization did not rely solely on the index for its arson prevention program. It supplemented the data with street surveys, word-of-mouth, and organizers' knowledge. The organization saw the arson problem as not just a building problem but an owner problem, an attempt to harass occupants to leave and make way for future gentrification of the area. This interpretation, however, was difficult to convey to government authorities and commercial insurance companies in order to ensure preventive actions. The effectiveness of computer data was limited by the social, political, and economic situation in which it was used.

Whatever the limits of its predictive efficiency or political effectiveness, the index was used as an organizing tool, along with other computer-assisted information development. As a result, tenant groups were formed and, with sufficient group pressure, were able to force enforcement of building codes or even, through supportive state law, the vesting of ownership in tenant governance. Here then, organized pressure, within an at least a nominally supportive legal structure, made computer data effective through mobilizing community pressure to get policymakers' attention.

However, arson and other neighborhood problems are not likely to be much improved without better access to authorities for community people to ensure policy enforcement and the resources for community development.

In each of these instances of policy, environmental, and community activism, information alone was not enough to produce change. Communication, organization, and advocacy were part of the equation. All these elements were far more accessible and effective because they were enabled with IT tools.

IT Support Groups

Very few organizations in disadvantaged areas have the technological or human information technology infrastructure to use the potential for building health-supporting communities that lies in the organized use of information technology. Acknowledging this, a variety of IT support groups, mainly staffed by volunteers, have sprung up in some cities across the country, from Boston to Portland to Canada (Johnson 1984; Nirv 1991; Miller 1993).

One New York group helped community-based, nonprofit groups find funds to buy IT equipment and, with its 150 volunteers, offered technical assistance through training workshops, redistribution of donated equipment, and services in special interest areas such as computers and disabilities, church-based programs, shelters and soup kitchens, job training, and education (Malbin 1991).

The experience of these support groups suggests the importance of working closely with local people not only to customize the IT systems to their particular circumstances, but also to tailor training and ongoing troubleshooting support to the rapid staff turnover that is common in small local groups. Small groups often lack incentives to fully use their new IT capacity when publicly available data are not in useful forms and when officials are reluctant to release their data. In these instances, IT support groups can sometimes play a mediating role in obtaining, transforming, and shaping the data to the needs of community groups (Bernstein 1991; Cordero 1991).

Public Services

Governments have been rapidly wiring themselves since the early 1980s. Nearly all cities of over 10,000 people had at least in-house computerized information systems by the end of the decade. By 1990 there were ten times as many personal computers for city employees as there were five years earlier (King and Kraemer 1991). The purpose was efficiency and cost control for office operations. But beyond that, cities began to move toward direct service delivery—of welfare payments, customer inquiries for utility bills and tax bills, citizen complaints, 24-hour access to the mayor's office, and information about government services to citizens. City governments also reached out to other governments with electronic networks to share information and experiences on common issues (King and Kraemer 1991).

Government electronic networks are common throughout the affluent world, but wiring occurred more rapidly where central governments provided technical assistance and other incentives to encourage local jurisdictions to develop their electronic capacity. That support did not exist in the United States until the early nineties (King and Kraemer 1991).

The wiring of American cities was primarily driven by state and local governments' search for efficiency in their administration and services. In this, they met with some successes (Hoff and Stormgaard 1991). In California, a dozen electronic kiosks, comparable to automated teller machines, were placed in convenient public sites like malls, markets, and libraries. They presented a "single face to government," a user-friendly, topic-based menu of employment, education, health care, legal, business, and government services. The information was available in both English and Spanish, with audio and visual guidance and a touch screen.

People used each kiosk 36 times a day, approaching 300,000 times in the two-year test. The vast majority found them easy to use and felt better prepared to contact government offices; over half said the machines saved them from any further contact with a government office. Items such as birth certificates and licenses could be had by using a credit card; the item was then mailed to the consumer. Viewed as a success, the state-sponsored system was to be expanded to all localities (Hinton 1993).

At the federal level, with the thrust toward "reinventing government" under the Clinton administration, all agencies were to "reengineer," to rethink how they could best carry out their mission. Plans were to cover strategy and operations, service delivery, technology, human resources, and facilities, incorporating IT to the maximum feasible extent.

A study of the Social Security Administration (SSA), among the best such agency in the world, showed that it did not take full advantage of the new technologies (OTA 1994). The study suggested that because more than 20 percent of older households have computers, the agency should consider an on-line program to supply beneficiaries with SSA resources, such as publications and data lists; tools, such as applications forms; transaction capabilities allowing address changes and account information; and specialized instructions for special groups, such as preretirees and disabled people.

Going beyond the individual "customer," the Office of Technology Assessment, which conducted the study, recommended that SSA give higher priority to funding the involvement of grass roots groups in electronic services delivery and the development of community infrastructure (such as libraries and senior centers) to enable them to directly deliver electronic SSA services or to act as intermediaries. It also proposed that the agency create and join other federal and state agencies in designing on-line directories and "one-stop shopping" sites for integrated electronic services, such as health and employment, which would be accessible by "smart cards" or other methods.

In some places local governments went beyond a self- or service-oriented emphasis and extended their electronic net in ways that allowed citizens to act independently as well as in partnership with their governors, as the following case demonstrates.

References

Benton Foundation. 1994. *Universal Services and the Information Superhighway*. Washington, DC: The Benton Foundation.

Bernstein, B. 1991. "Microcomputers in Political Campaigns: Lessons from the Jackson Campaign in New York." *Computers in Human Services* 8 (1): 55–70.

Cook, R. 1985. "Predicting Arson." *Byte* (August): 239–45.

Cordero, A. 1991. "Computers and Community Organizing: Issues and Examples from New York City." *Computers in Human Services* 1: 89–104.

Furger, R. 1992. "Consumer Watch." *PC World* (September): 27–29.

General Accounting Office (GAO). 1991. *EPA'S Toxic Release Inventory Is Useful but Can Be Improved*. Washington, DC: U.S. Congress.

Groups and Associations Membership. 1988. Unpublished Report. Simmons Market Research Bureau, Washington, DC.

Hinton, P. 1993. "INFO/CALIFORNIA: Pilot Project Analysis." 1993. Sacramento, CA: Health and Welfare Agency Data Center.

Hoff, J., and K. Stormgaard. 1991. "Information Technology Between Citizen and Administration." *Informatization and the Public Sector* 1 (3): 213–35.

King, J. L., and K. L. Kraemer. 1991. "Patterns of Success in Municipal Information Systems: Lessons from US Experience." *Informatization and the Public Sector* 1 (1): 21–39.

Ladd, E. 1989. *The American Policy: The People and Their Government*. New York: W. W. Norton.

Lynn, F., and A. Koebrick. 1992. "Toxics Release Inventory. Environmental Democracy in Action." Report. Washington, DC: EPA Office of Toxic Substances.

MacLean, A., and P. Orum. 1992. *Progress Report: Community Right-to-Know*. Washington, DC: Working Group on Community Right-to-Know.

Malbin, J. 1991. "Computers for Community Service." *NYPC Magazine* (September): 37–38.

Miller, P. 1993. "The Community Computer Movement." *CPSR Newsletter* 11 (3): 6–8.

National Public Telecomputing Network (NPTN). 1993. *The Bluebook*. Cleveland, OH: NPTN.

Nirv Community Resource Centre. 1991. Web. Program description. Toronto, Ontario: Web.

Office of Disease Prevention and Health Promotion. 1994. "Level of Interest in Public Policy Issues." Unpublished Preliminary Survey Data. Washington, DC: U.S. Public Health Service.

Office of Technology Assessment (OTA). 1990. "Critical Connections: Communication for the Future." Washington, DC: U.S. Congress.

———. 1994. *Social Security Administration's Decentralized Computer Strategy: Issues and Options*. Washington, DC: U.S. Congress, April.

Ornstein, N., et al. 1988. *The People, the Press, and Politics*. New York: Addison-Wesley.

Roth, E. 1987. "Power Surge in Personal Computers." *Editorial Research Reports* 6 (9 January).

Settina, N., and P. Orum. 1991. *Making the Difference, II: More Uses of Right-to-Know in the Fight Against Toxics*. Washington, DC: Center for Policy Alternatives and Working Group on Community Right-To-Know.

Taxpayer Assets Project. 1993. *Crown Jewels Campaign*. Information Policy Note. Washington, DC, 2 October.

CHAPTER

13

GIVING VOICE TO THE VOICELESS IN WESTSUN

The Homeless Find a Place in Cyberspace

THE SMALL, rather self-satisfied city of Westsun on the West Coast was once known as a haven for 1960s left-of-center politics. In the nineties, its affluent and largely liberal citizens have wondered whether it is becoming "Skid Row-by-the-Sea." In recent years homeless people have become ubiquitous in the streets and green spaces, curiously integrated into the life of the community, despite complaints from increasingly impatient and cost-conscious taxpayers.

Crowds of the homeless gathered twice a day in front of city hall, lining up for a meal served from a table set up to apportion the basics—stews, chili, or hot dogs, fresh or cooked veggies, fruit, bread, donuts or cakes—a potluck of unsold produce from local merchants. Serving mainly older and young men, the atmosphere was generally quiet and the surroundings kept tidy and cleared after the event. The only exception was an older woman, living in a mental and physical world of her own, who made her abode adjacent to the city hall entrance, along with her dog, cot, and supermarket cart containing all her belongings. Some said these reminders of the city's problems were allowed full public view as a way to compel an adequate approach to the problem of homelessness, to keep it on the public agenda of decision makers and taxpayers.

Only a few yards away from this site, through the city hall entrance and behind a dark-glass, air-conditioned enclosed space that houses Westsun's mainframe computer, were the offices of the city's information systems department. There a link was created between reformers and the homeless issue, between social advocacy and information technology, another picture of community information technology.

A Haven for the Favored

Westsun attracted homeless people and others not only because of its hospitable weather and shoreline, but because of its citizens, almost

100,000 in all. The residents were relatively young, living either with small families or as singles in well-appointed rented housing made affordable by very well paid professional and managerial jobs. Overall, they were much better educated, healthier, and allowed far less poverty to persist in their community than in the rest of their state or the nation (Bureau of the Census 1988).

The state, although wealthier than most of the nation as a whole, was among the less generous with its more vulnerable people, including young children living in poverty. It gave them poorer access to basic health care, although it had an abundance of physicians. A third of its students did not finish high school, although it had some of the best educational institutions in the country. Crime and unemployment were big problems even though its cities and industries were enviable. Its environmental problems were among the worst, in spite of its renowned beauty (APHA 1992). In the nineties, it also had the unenviable record of the largest shortage of affordable rental housing in the nation. Twice as many low-income families needed housing than the available supply, according to a Westsun city council task force report.

The Political Agenda

It was not just their favored lifestyle that made Westsunners different and made their city a haven for the homeless. It was their strong sense of community, the mutual trust and presumption of good intentions even among rivals. In the eighties, a slate of young activists got themselves elected to the city council on a platform of strict rent control and participatory democracy—"in an age of low voter turnout, media manipulation of elections, and widespread public distrust of politicians." This liberal majority enacted its promises, using citizen advisory commissions, a system of neighborhood organizations, and training for public access cable television. Public monies were invested in public art, libraries, children, elders, and bilingual services, and upgrading the environment.

Yet these electoral and policy successes brought problems in the 1990s, among them a housing shortage. Landlords refused to improve their apartments and were not allowed to convert them to condominiums. Homeowner neighborhood associations protested the visibility of homeless strangers. The problems of environmental pollution, regional in nature, brought mandated changes from state government, making demands not only on the city budget, but also on lifestyles. A four-day government work week was ordered to save energy costs and the air. For all this, councilors received $50 a month, a reasonable salary when it began in the 1940s. But campaigning for office now cost $250,000.

There were, however, other compensations, not least the capacity to influence and bring about changes to which council members and aspirants were personally committed. And, the council was among the first to use, from the early 1980s, a new set of tools for governance—information technology. By the early 1990s, each councilor had personal computers and laser printers, as well as voice mail at the office and at home, a laptop computer, and a car phone.

By the end of the eighties, the main local political issues were neighborhood protection and affordable housing, both tied to homelessness. According to the mayor, himself once a tenant organizer and founder of a local nonprofit housing corporation:

> This problem is beginning to polarize our city. We haven't understood all the implications of our programs. . . . We have to collectively search for the best combinations of policies and programs for solutions that are respectful of the rights of all people, including homeless people. But we must also be cognizant of the public safety concerns that have been evident in the community. . . . The escalating violence in the parks is related to the drug trade. . . . The dealers have been hiding among the homeless population.

The dreams of participatory public decision making were also clouded, as the mayor noted:

> Unless we have strong limits on campaign contributions and seriously consider other reforms, such as districting, we're going to continue to see decisions made at the council level which aren't in the best interests of residents, but are in the interests of those making money on commercial development.

The Push toward Information Technology

Regional and state pressures increased as public fiscal deficits grew deeper and jobs less secure. The state mandated controls on expenditures, environmental pollution, and traffic. This forced innovative changes in public and private "workstyles," including the use of public access computer terminals to provide county services information to citizens and the development of "telecommuting" for county employees. Employees were provided with computers at home or a satellite office to shorten travel time, reduce fuel use and noxious emissions, and improve productivity and job satisfaction. The state and region were drawing on IT to help address some complex and long-term problems.

When Westsun's governors became early adopters of IT almost ten years before the mandates came down, some were dubious. Computers were too expensive or would be too time-consuming to learn to use. However, once tutored, they became converted and competent users.

Then in the mid-1980s, came an opportunity to open their electronic system to Westsun citizens. One of the conservative minority on the council, a "workaholic," initiated the step. He informally asked the information systems department whether his computer could be networked to others' outside city government so that he could contact them after hours. The department gave an unenthusiastic, "we'll look into it" response, hoping to decline at a later date and not wanting to address the technical and other complexities involved.

Feasibility

Exploratory discussions began at a leisurely pace between the information systems department and experts from the local private university that used city hall assignments to train graduate students. The pace picked up after a large commercial developer who had brought both wealth and controversy to the community (in fact, he was known variously as opportunist, liberal, and patron of local arts) went before the council to request council agendas and staff reports from its network through public access electronic mail (e-mail). Such information could assist his own lobbying efforts. The council then instructed the information systems department to study city communications and report back on the feasibility of public access to electronic information.

There was no question of *technical* feasibility, but was a public information network (PIN) something that the public wanted? A university survey showed surprisingly great interest, and that a third of Westsunners owned computers, three times the national average.

The Public Information Network

What might a PIN try to do? The proposed purposes followed the implied wishes of the council and those gleaned from the public survey, as well as the liberal inclinations of the academic advisers:

- Provide electronic access to public information by city residents and workers
- Provide an alternative means for the public to convey needs and preferences to local government and other residents
- Enhance the delivery and awareness of public services and facilitate the public service inquiry process
- Provide a forum for participation in issue discussions by residents to promote a sense of community
- Extend the opportunity to understand computer technology and offer access to equipment to learn to communicate through information technology.

To meet these aims the menu of available information and communication options contained an array of choices, such as extensive voter and electoral data, city notices, reports, agendas, and minutes, as well as information on 34 city departments and divisions, ranging from water services and conservation to construction regulations, consumer affairs, and fair housing rights. There were also modules containing services and activities of community programs, including libraries, neighborhood associations, cultural events, and a directory of all social services and educational programs. A "mailroom" gave the electronic addresses of all public officials, and a "conference" space allowed public discussion of any issue at the wish of any user, with dozens of topics eventually under discussion at any one time, from local to national problems, from science to sports.

Social Issues

Other issues of concern were the legal liability of the city, confidentiality, "unfair competition" to potential commercial networks by a taxpayer-supported network, and whether PIN would infringe on First Amendment free speech rights. Most of these issues were worked out in a simple agreement signed by registrants, with the city reserving the right to remove users from participation privileges if the contract were broken. It prohibited the conduct of illegal business on PIN or using it for commercial purposes.

Much of the "etiquette" and other social risks were to be treated in ways that occur in all public discourse, through gradual and mutual formation of unwritten rules and the comments of users among themselves. In addition, users had to use their own names (or the names they gave at registration), implying some control over "flaming" (using abusive speech).

The local American Civil Liberties Union chapter endorsed PIN as a vehicle promoting free speech. There was no "gatekeeper" to the system. It was for all who lived in the city. Subject matter had no limits, except that any new subject was designated by the interested parties to a labeled and separate conference.

In practice a wide and unfettered range of views sped across the terminal screens from liberals and conservatives. The conservative cause was led by a local leader whose opponents, as noted in the local press, "compare her to [Joseph] McCarthy, Nixon, and [David] Duke" while "her admirers compare her to Ralph Nader, Mother Teresa, and Rambo." The homeless and the wealthy joined nonvoters and the mayor, children and elders. But only those literate in English had access. This language restriction became a problem that PIN would address in the future. A program for teaching English-speaking nonreaders was added later as a partial answer.

Expectations

Before PIN began, elected officials saw it as a way to keep their "finger on the pulse" of the community. It was to be "a marketplace for ideas," a way to influence decisions, although not necessarily representative of the population. PIN would provide the public with information and knowledge, would support opinion formation, would identify like-minded people, and would thus encourage advocacy and participation in the political process.

Some city department bureaucrats were less enthusiastic. They feared they would receive more complaints. City law required every citizen complaint to be answered in a laborious process that took about two months. They were also reluctant to open their public records to a wider and perhaps more critical public. They felt "too exposed."

A very limited pilot test was done between the police department, which was an enthusiastic PIN supporter, and some Neighborhood Watch residents, who were not very computer literate. The purpose of this less-than-scientific experiment was viewed as basically political. The Information Systems Department knew that the council wanted a PIN system. The test was regarded a success, and the PIN proposal was approved without opposition. It was to be implemented by the department as soon as possible, but without any new funds or staff. That meant the Information Systems Department had to use its own resources and ingenuity to produce the program.

Resources at a Bargain

City hall and the state and local boards of education used the same large in-state IT producer as their supplier. The Information Systems Department quickly took advantage of this contact. It proposed a persuasive deal with the sales office: a donation of computers in return for national publicity about what was probably the first venture of its kind. The firm agreed to supply $350,000 in equipment. It also donated its own database management software, which became the basis for PIN's databases and another promotional point for sales, noted in company publications.

The IT producer had a donor unit that guided its grant programs, growing more than sevenfold over the 1980s to $61 million. Initially it did not publicize its donations, but finding such grants in public favor, it began to advertise them.

The information systems department also found a well-known network systems firm that agreed to contribute its technology. The firm began its self-promotion in several publications:

> Westsun is living up to its reputation as a progressive city. . . . Its PIN network, a unique experiment in government accessibility, has given residents an interactive link to City Hall. . . . One of its first decisions was that it should use the OURNET system. The City had never used OURNET before, but that didn't deter them because OURNET offered one characteristic no other operating system did—portability. "The reason we picked OURNET to do the PIN project is that we wanted to have it as transferable as possible to other vendors' hardware."

The information systems department then persuaded its software producer to donate a new programming package that the department staff had in any case wanted to learn.

Programmers from the department took about a year to integrate PIN components, develop the menus, and isolate the databases for the system. The system downloaded data from the city's mainframe computer to 15 public terminals, which increased to 35 within three years and could support 64 users at one time on public and personal computers in homes and offices. Terminals were placed in the city hall lobby, libraries, youth and senior centers, and elsewhere.

Registration

The city manager wanted an early and very public opening of the system to get full media coverage. The publicity gave a boost to user registration. To further inform Westsunners about PIN, along with printed handouts the information systems department produced a video and used the city's public access cable channel to discuss PIN. It also published an occasional newsletter to keep users abreast of changes and improvements in the system.

Training and Maintenance

The department managed the PIN system through designated PIN coordinators in each city office and at each site where public terminals were located. It trained them as facilitators on site. Most of the training for users, beyond the short manual given to all registrants, was done by the department on a flexible basis. In addition to answering individual questions about PIN on e-mail, trainers held sessions of about 1.5 hours for about eight people, repeated several times a day over a period of several days, including evenings and Saturdays. These sessions rotated through selected sites every four to six months.

Another maintenance chore, one *not* routinized, was updating the databases and notices, and posting the minutes from the council meetings. There was little systematic effort to discover why some sites did not use PIN very much while others did, except to observe that changes of personnel sometimes preceded a drop in usage, suggesting the need for monitoring and ongoing staff training.

Responses to PIN

Because the program was one of the first of its kind, and in spite of educated guesses, no one knew what the actual reaction to PIN would be.

The City Departments

Where some city bureaucrats were wary of PIN before it began, many changed their views afterward. For example, as the cable TV management unit responded to queries and complaints, public attitudes about its competence improved rapidly; viewers were more accepting of the cable system service, whether or not their individual complaints were resolved.

The police department was especially responsive to PIN users, led by its new chief who was on the local college Futures Automation Committee. "Computers and their applications are a long term interest of mine," he said. "I strongly believe in the 'high-tech, high-touch' approach to law enforcement. . . . People like the idea that the police use PIN to listen to them." However, the public did not actually report crimes or suspicious activity on PIN, which the department had hoped would help them track patterns and target vulnerable locales.

Unlike police leadership, the response by some staff officers was that PIN was a nuisance. They were "not receptive to what they call the 'touchy-feely' aspect of police work."

Bureaucratic Users

After more than two years of experience with PIN, the information systems department surveyed about half of the city departments to get their views on the system. Contrary to expectations, public complaints took up only a quarter of their messages; most were general queries and requests for services, and occasionally compliments.

City personnel thought that PIN increased interdepartmental services and improved response time. Although it did not necessarily improve relations with the public, they believed it would be an increasingly important communications and democratizing tool for the future. PIN made their work more interesting, even when it increased their workload. It helped them be more responsive to public concerns, especially about the city and its plans, and the issue of homelessness. Most thought that the most important parts of PIN were the communications services—that is, the e-mail and discussion forums, rather than the information services, such as bulletin boards, calendars, and services listings.

Tallies of actual use by city personnel showed that most were passive users. They read their e-mail, and about half read some of the discussions and bulletin boards. Fewer than half initiated e-mail or posted their own messages. In general, then, PIN seemed a probably worthwhile and increasingly necessary innovation, but not one about which city staff were very enthusiastic, still being uncertain about what it might mean for their own jobs.

Elected Officials

Council members answered queries in their own e-mail, as any prudent elected representative would. Initially, many joined in the conference discussions. Some became highly vocal about their experience with PIN.

One conservative member who participated actively in the conferences, announced publicly after more than a year that she was quitting PIN because she was "fed up with being the target of mean, snotty, political attacks" by "people who pound out their anger on their keyboard."

Some councilors read the conferences but did not give public replies because PIN users "hold your feet to the fire." Others avoided PIN debates out of fear of exposing themselves. As one council member noted, "I think that one of the issues is whether you want to put yourself out there and be subject to criticism, or be proven wrong. . . . PIN is time-consuming. . . . We don't have the staff to put into it. It's scary to get involved in some conferences." Two officials "got fed up with the conference because of vituperative name calling" concerning their positions on zoning.

But there were those who logged on every day and were not concerned about public responses. They were just thrilled their constituents were talking. A few used the system to put out fact-filled essays that triggered debates and got responses to proposals.

Nonlocal Politicians

PIN attempted to provide Westsunners with electronic access to their state and federal representatives. State legislators, known to be liberal, participatory democrats, declined to accept an e-mail address, pleading staff time problems.

The congressional representative, considered a liberal, accepted the invitation and proclaimed to his constituents that he was

> the first Member of Congress to go on-line with his constituents. . . . PIN demonstrates how computers can be used to facilitate greater communication between elected officials and their constituents. It will allow me to do a better job of serving my constituents and provide an important new channel of communication.

In practice, the representative's district office staff either answered PIN queries on his behalf or, more often, sent them to Washington, DC, for research and reply. This often took several weeks, frustrating PIN users. Users also did not like the fact that their congressman did not personally enter the conference discussions. The staff felt they had to do time-consuming work for only a few constituents.

City Hall's Image

Regardless of the views of individuals in government or the effectiveness of PIN for government efficiency and participatory democracy, the general message to the public was rendered by the press in terms that pleased PIN's sponsors. The image created by the national media in front page stories was glowing:

> Declaring itself "the city of the future," Westsun has activated a new computer network that puts a storehouse of information . . . at the fingertips of city residents. . . . Questions and complaints can be computer-messaged to City Hall. . . . Westsun will be a pioneer in the use of interactive computer networks to enable the public to communicate with government. . . . [the donor suppliers are] hoping that this will be a showpiece leading to sales elsewhere.

City hall welcomed dozens of visitors and inquiries from around the world, and received awards for good government (for promoting consumer advocacy through its grievance information services) and for technology innovation (from one of its hardware donor companies).

Outside City Hall

The sites where PIN's public terminals were installed used the system for improving services and achieving organizational purposes. In other places there was an utter lack of interest. Among the most active groups were the better-organized and educated environmental groups. But in the Senior Recreation Center, the terminal was left mainly unused on a corner table, as elders mingled and talked, had a snack, or played cards with each other. Why use a computer to communicate when you could do better face-to-face? What many of them would have liked was not possible on PIN: "Can I talk to my doctor on this [terminal]?"

The Library

At the other end of the spectrum of PIN users, the library system put PIN to work for several tasks. It answered specific questions on-line about literally almost anything in the world and beyond, and did so within 24 hours. The staff used interlibrary e-mail to work among themselves. They took public suggestions about library policies and, where possible, made changes. In a strategic sense, the library used e-mail comments to justify its requests for budget changes and used the discussion forum as a sounding board to get public feedback on proposed changes in library services. The PIN terminals were kept visible and promoted with signs, brochures, and personal assistance.

Neighborhood Support Center

The Neighborhood Support Center had one of the public access PIN terminals. It was a rather unusual nonprofit organization, established under city law as an independent entity to provide support for community participation. Rather than having each community group seek direct funding from the council, which had led to charges of political favoritism, the center provided a centralized staff to support eligible neighborhood organizations.

The neighborhood groups were geographically based, democratically organized, multipurpose, and nonpolitical units covering most of Westsun's neighborhoods. Their agendas dealt mainly with housing and homelessness, land use, and the environment. Some had high goals—for example, "to strengthen our sense of community and to share it with a growing number of our neighbors." The center offered these groups information on city issues, notices of pending policy and development projects and assistance in responding to them, community outreach and ombudsman services, a newsletter, logistical support for meetings, and training for volunteers.

The center itself used PIN in a limited way, sometimes obtaining city staff reports, communicating with city hall, using the directories to refer individuals and groups to available services, and reading the electronic forums on crime, recreation, and housing and development. It found PIN was an indirect benefit when its own constituents, the neighborhood groups, used it themselves, thereby saving center staff time.

But the groups did not use PIN regularly. Other low-budget, nonprofit community service groups, such as the Drop-In Center for the Homeless, rarely used PIN. The center thought low-income people and groups had little time to learn about or use PIN and that their educational background precluded any inclination to go to PIN.

One exception was Newstart, a new group partly financed by the city to work with young people. It used the center's PIN terminal for its own information and communication purposes. Working with the police department in an antidrug program, it taught kids to use a PIN terminal in a neighborhood police-sponsored youth center. Newstart also showed them how to send messages to their counterparts at the city's special "continuation" high school, Pinnacle High, which shared its expertise with the youth center.

Pinnacle High School

The students at Pinnacle were "dropouts" who returned to a special, individualized, self-paced curriculum designed around their own talents and interests. About a third of them, under the tutelage of a skilled instructor, used PIN along with a wide spectrum of other information technologies: compact discs, VCRs, and powerful personal computers and printers with complex programs. On-line, the students discussed the homeless issue. Their views, like those of adults, ranged from "throw them out" to sympathy for "poor people." Other topics included getting birth control on campus, planning the school yearbook, smoking on campus, and censorship. As a school tool PIN had much to offer from the educator's point of view:

> Airing their [students'] opinions in a public forum forced them to defend those positions when their peers gave them some heat. . . . Many students who had been rather shy about expressing themselves in public found their voice on e-mail. . . . Students loved finding a note in their [electronic] mailbox. . . . Well-thought-out questions came from students in e-mail that might not have received the attention they deserved in class. . . . Students began to address questions and comments to the school principal and received personal answers.

In the eyes of an educator, "PIN is most effective when knowledge and power people use it," providing "experiences of value" for public users. But the leaders in Westsun's education system had "not bitten" because, as with some elected officials, they feared electronic attacks. School board members were "no longer willing to post messages on PIN," wary of political exposure.

PIN and the Public

Individual Users

After two years in operation, PIN's more than 3,000 registered users looked overall like the "typical" citizens of Westsun: adults under 50, well educated and earning about $50,000 a year in professional or managerial work. Most had access to a computer at home or at work. But by the second year, there was a 50 percent increase in those who used public terminals. Access to PIN increased by half in the second year, averaging about 1,500 communications a week, with 50 communications going directly to city hall.

Three-quarters of the users were readers. They were passive users like city personnel and elected officials. The most often used PIN services by far were messaging, e-mail, and conferencing. Only a quarter of the log ons were bulletin board–based information. As pointed out by Westsun's leading conservative, "People do not crave new sources of information so much as new venues for talking to one another."

The information systems department's research also confirmed what most observers knew anecdotally. The lion's share of PIN use came from a core group of about 50 to 90 people who logged on from once a week to twice daily. Much of this use was for discussion of current political issues. These users were thought by some to be dominating the discussions, engaging in "metacommentary" by commenting on others' ways of commenting, rather than making comments themselves.

Virtual Organizations

The on-screen activity also spun off community activity, "virtual" electronic organizations capable of action in the real world. In one contentious local issue, the entrepreneur who first requested a public electronic network wanted to rezone land to build a hotel. He wanted most of it for commercial development rather than the accepted 50/50 public-private split. In response, an on-line campaign began that eventually resulted in the 50/50 choice. It also led to the loss of a pro-development councilor's seat, which she had held for 15 years.

Another longer-lasting virtual organization became a face-to-face group as some users shared their "concern that PIN had not yet appealed to more people." The group met to develop suggestions on how to improve the quality of the system and attract more users. This ad hoc group on PIN became in effect an advisory committee to the information systems department, which welcomed and used its suggestions.

PIN Action

The most visible and active group, one with many spin-offs, was the PIN Action Group. The issue that brought the group into being was homelessness. PIN was the medium that made organization possible, providing an economical way to gain political support for government action.

Before PIN, Westsun's parks department had shown no interest in constructing showers and lockers in its parks for use by the public, including the homeless, which was an idea suggested by a well-regarded Westsun resident. The issue was too controversial. But when the resident raised the idea in a PIN on-line conference on homelessness, "people loved it"—including many who were regarded as conservatives. Political leaders were still wary, especially as highly conservative "demagogues" began to organize against it on PIN.

Within three months the PIN Action Group was meeting face-to-face. A core group of 12 to 20 people, including both "homed" and homeless people, called on a variety of experts in the government and community to write a proposal. "The comments of the homeless were invaluable in this whole process because we wouldn't have known where to focus [without them]," one group member remarked.

The homeless people who became involved in the group offered these insights on-line:

- People see me on PIN not as a stupid, lazy bum, but someone equal to them. . . . I have met people that I would probably have never met even if I was sheltered.
- I try to look good, not homeless. . . . Thank you for letting me stay in the library and use PIN during the day.
- On weekends the drop-in centers are closed, and also the Salvation Army is closed Saturday, and I think only sandwiches are served Sunday morning. So especially with Sunday (no city hall lawn meal that day), weekends are short on meals.
- Do those people who do serve meals check them for adequate nutrition—enough protein offered, vitamin C, etc.? And regarding nutrition, I sometimes wonder if those persons exhibiting bad behavior may be doing so in large part due to a nutritional lack that has brought frustration. . . . Has anyone particularly noticed. . . . several homeless women beyond middle age? They seem to be really suffering, and they are older persons. What can someone come up with that would assist these persons? Sometimes with homeless women it takes a certain skill or knack to approach them, to come near, or to get them to take some aid and getting around dignity or pride refusals. I have often wondered if someday some sisters from a woman's group would go out periodically, meet these women, and try to resolve their poverty.
- I have experience being homeless, and have done research especially in the legal area: discrimination and civil rights. I am available to meet with people, and to make friends. Please contact me by PIN.

SHLOCK

The PIN Action Group submitted its proposal to the council. Coded SHLOCK for its emphasis on public showers and lockers, it also proposed vouchers to allow homeless people to use laundromats. At the urging of its homeless members, the group added job counseling and training resources, bus fare and lunch money, and the development of a job bank, a computerized, PIN-based listing of local jobs to be available in all social service agencies and community service sites.

While city staff examined the plan, PIN Action attempted private fund-raising, getting $5,000 from a used goods sale and a donation of 30 lockers from a local manufacturer. They also negotiated with community groups and laundry facilities, which were not enthusiastic to manage or accept vouchers from homeless people.

Throughout a year of planning and negotiating, ideas and methods were debated on PIN, for all the public to see, to learn about, and to engage in. However, recognizing that both potential allies and adversaries were watching, and not wanting to expose their political strategy before the fact, the group continued to meet face-to-face for strategic planning.

Faced with SHLOCK, the council first sought a feasibility study and then approved installation of the shower facilities and lockers. This was decided in the larger context of an election, and the urgent issue of affordable housing was debated in view of tightening budgets. PIN and the Action Group were seen by elected officials as a spur to community interest in Westsun's Task Force on Homelessness and the subsequent public hearings that would help the council decide its priorities for larger housing policy and budget issues.

The PIN Action Group obtained membership on the task force, and several activists, both "homed and homeless," presented testimony at well-attended public hearings. They pressed the issue of affordable housing, recommending means to finance its development, as well as job banks and SHLOCK services, public education, community involvement, and public safety for all citizens. All of their ideas found expression in the task force recommendations.

SHLOCK in the Real World

In the end, the council's support for the original SHLOCK proposal itself amounted to $106,000 to install ten showers. The vouchers were managed by one community center, which issued them three times a week, and were accepted by one laundromat during slack hours. The job bank began slowly at the community center, its software developed by one of PIN Action Group's formerly homeless members. The group recruited graduate students to survey local employers for job openings, giving the students course credits for their efforts. The group also trained volunteers as job counselors to assist in job finding, work transition, and temporary housing. In the first three months, the program counseled about 15 people a week and placed one person in a job.

It was clear that the job bank idea was not viable unless the city accepted responsibility for its development. The action group itself could not sustain it, nor even develop its potential. The group continued to meet on-line to monitor and urge progress on its own ideas and the wider issues advocated by the Task Force on Homelessness, which could institutionalize what the Action Group had begun.

PIN Women

In PIN's early days, its active participants were men, who outnumbered women on the system by about 10 to 1. After two years the ratio was about 2 to 1. Women's initial reaction to PIN was based on their mutual awareness of sexist comments in the discussions, which deterred their participation. This commonality brought them together in several breakfast meetings to develop a supporting "joint front" on PIN.

Calling themselves PIN WOMEN, they subsequently proceeded on-line with discussions of such issues as access to abortion services. This caught the eye of a councilwoman who, after a meeting with the group, had one of them named to Westsun's Women's Commission. Eventually, three PIN WOMEN were among the nine commissioners, including the chair. One of their first moves was to have the commission go on-line on PIN with its own agenda, minutes, reports, mail service, and forum.

Prospects and Plans

In spite of a tight city budget, all agreed that PIN would slowly and steadily expand. It would not only inform people about where and how to get public services through new county information databases, but would also supply many services on-line—for example, applications for library cards and books and forms for licenses and complaints, in friendlier and more graphic formats.

The system would also become more educational. Through an agreement with a local community college, it would offer a series of on-line lectures on a variety of everyday and academic topics from auto mechanics to history. The lectures would be followed by conferences and question-answer sessions with the instructor. There would be space for classroom projects to encourage students to use PIN as an information resource, or to have, for example, a journalism class collaborate in a joint project with a newspaper. The college would also list volunteer tutors in several areas of expertise, allowing students of any age to call on them on-line in a private conference. Finally, there would be arrangements for closed conferences for particular organizations, such as the Museum Society.

In this educational joint venture, both parties would gain more than the costs of their contributions. The network expansion to news organizations would obviously improve PIN, give it more visibility, and attract a wider public. The information systems department would provide the necessary network training and system maintenance, as well as documentation and publicity for the new services.

The community college would benefit through the educational and research possibilities for its students and faculty, through "distance education," thereby attracting a new student group that could enroll in credit-giving, tuition-based courses. As importantly, in an era of cutbacks in educational budgets, the college would be seen as being relevant and responsive to the community that was supporting it.

However, goodwill among community organizations ran up against barriers that good intentions alone could not overcome. Technologically, for example, PIN's interest in reaching the seniors of Westsun might be possible by attracting them with SeniorNet. But discussions between the Information Systems Department and SeniorNet showed that such a program would need a minimum of $25,000 in start-up funds. Even expansion to educational institutions, whether Pinnacle High, the community college, universities, or elsewhere, required new telephone lines or other more complex and costly technological changes. Just the addition of more public terminals at more convenient sites—laundromats, recreation centers, major supermarkets—and easier registration at libraries and public agencies would compete with other priorities for limited funds.

It was not difficult to think of new ways to give the public more reason to get on-line. The hard part was finding the resources to do the job, even in the favored community of Westsun.

Summary: Social Climate, Social Questions, Collective Conclusions

Looking from the outside, Westsun appeared to have far more of the good life than most American cities: natural and constructed beauty; an affluent, industrious, well-educated and engaged citizenry; a record of caring for its more vulnerable members. At the same time, it shared a condition with others who turned to information technology as a new set of tools to serve their purposes. Westsun, first in city hall, then within segments of the public, wanted to do better what it was doing—connecting with constituencies—and wanted to face new problems—homelessness—with limited resources.

Far more than most, the city had all essential ingredients for initiating community IT in the form of a public information network (PIN): elected leaders with a demonstrable history of participatory governance; the paid time of competent staff and of interested, idea-prone citizens with a recent history of community cooperation; and technical, managerial, and strategic expertise to arrange the IT and the organizational structure, and to get agreement by council, community groups, and contributors of hardware and software.

In Westsun, all this could be done with few new dollars. It did require strategic timing, targeting familiar entrepreneurial contacts and others, and negotiating skill to array for them more gains than losses in sales, image building, future ties, and celebrating First Amendment rights. The same program, if ventured elsewhere, would have required searching for funds, contacts, expertise, and facilities, and would probably have been done on volunteer, patchwork time through trial and error, taking much longer and perhaps failing at any discouraging juncture along the way.

Westsun had other assets that were critical to PIN's successful initiation and operation. Regardless of the personal views and early reactions of city staff and council users, PIN as government policy for the future was accepted as a fact of political life, and all welcomed the city's capacity to project itself as a leader in high-tech participatory democracy. City hall had access to local and national mass media, its own public access cable channel, and technology for video and other media production, as well as the interest of its commercial suppliers in publicizing their contributions.

More than these supports, PIN could be managed by designating on-site staff in each unit to serve as IT coordinators to update users about changes in the system and to answer their questions. Where this mundane but essential service was absent, as in some of the community locations, the use of PIN fell off. When PIN worked smoothly, even skeptical users began to change their views of its usefulness. An added asset was the volunteer citizen group that monitored system problems and could suggest improvements to the information systems department.

In Westsun doubts about PIN persisted in city personnel and elected officials who worried about what it would mean for their job security. For department staff, could it mean replacement? For some councilors, state, and federal representatives, and local school board members, there seemed to be too high a political cost, with PIN exposing them to controversy and the implicit threat of loss at the next election. Their ideology, liberal or conservative, did not determine their participation; rather, it was the potential impact of PIN on their interests.

At the same time, PIN's value to local officials was apparent. Most of them monitored selected electronic discussions even when they decided not to participate. Some found a middle way by supplying information that was unknown to the discussants; a few simply reveled in democracy.

PIN's use at the community-based terminals depended, not surprisingly, on how easily it could provide information and communication services that people needed and could not get elsewhere. Part of making it easy was having the equipment visible, accessible, with very friendly instructions and nearby immediate personal help if necessary. These conditions were not met for elders who were not homebound. But politically and technologically sophisticated environmental and other public interest groups, the libraries, and some teachers found a good fit with PIN. Their background and experience had prepared them to use and adapt it to their own purposes. They used PIN not only for information and communication for their services and management tasks, but also to venture in new directions, involving their clientele, whether readers or pupils, in shaping the direction of their programs.

But other organizations, the low-budget community groups serving less advantaged people, did not have comparable experience and expectations, or the education or time to teach themselves about PIN. Much more support in the form of organized training, on-site staff time, demonstration of relevance, and perhaps software changes might have made PIN more enticing.

Yet, among the general public, there were indications of a change among users. After the first year, the public access terminals were increasingly used, especially by people whose education and jobs had not necessarily prepared them for IT, those who did not have personal computers at home and were not high-income earners. In addition, although among the public as in city hall, there were about three electronic readers to every writer, PIN users were going beyond seeking information and communication, beyond building a sense of "virtual community." They began to create organizations, "virtual organizations," electronic groups that were cohesive enough to have influence and take action in the face-to-face world. One of the most active was the PIN Action Group, which eventually became a formally incorporated organization whose "homed and homeless" members had a significant influence on Westsun's programs for addressing homelessness issues.

PIN as an organizing medium allowed users to become aware of each other and to communicate and come together on a relatively equal basis with their peers or opposites—homeless people, homeowners, conservatives, liberals, young people, women. Their effectiveness as a group thereafter depended on whether they had other requisites for organized action, beyond communication, information, and coordination, such as agreement on actionable goals, a means for guidance and accountability, and time and funds for action.

Lacking a sustainable base for these other organizational essentials, PIN Action could not itself easily enact its homeless support program, which became a precursor to future city-supported programs. These limits, inherent in nonprofit organizations, were why PIN Action focused on changing city housing policy rather than simply seeking a time-limited grant.

The fact that city policy supported PIN meant that the network, although it would be buffeted by budget shifts, would be sustained and grow, if slowly. It would become easier for more members of the community to join their counterparts as listeners and voices, and as actors in building community in the net and on the ground.

References

American Public Health Association (APHA). 1992. *Public Health Report Card*. Washington, DC: APHA.

Bureau of the Census. 1988. *County and City Data Book*. Washington, DC: U.S. Department of Commerce.

SECTION E

Some Lessons from the Cases

Where is the wisdom we have lost in knowledge? Where is the knowledge we have lost in information?

T. S. Eliot, *The Rock*

CHAPTER

14

CONNECTING THE CASES

Common Problems, Processes, and Impacts

IN THE predawn of the twenty-first century, the vistas are all too familiar: five localities, four small-to-moderate U.S. cities—Midwest, South, West Coast, an English country town. They all were impelled to change their ways during the eighties and nineties by the spillover of national economic and social problems onto state and municipal budgets and local troubles. Whether among Westsun's affluent, highly educated, high-tech-using activists, the church community in Southcity, or the aging natives of Hill Park, disadvantaged groups were growing because of job loss, homelessness, poverty, undereducation, and pollution. Limited funds and eroding political capital prevented adequate fiscal outlays from supporting public and private agency action. Yet the festering conditions bred more costly acute problems: infant mortality, teen pregnancy, substance abuse, AIDS, and unsafe environments heaped upon the mushrooming of chronic disease.

But new resources also entered the case portraits deriving from nationwide and global trends and from the diverse settings in which they were located. New options became available from emerging information technologies. Each site initiated an innovation in "community IT," the organized application of information technology to promote conditions supportive of community well-being and health, especially among economically disadvantaged groups. How they developed community IT, the problems they faced, and the strategies they used to deal with them suggest the kinds of policy support that are needed to make them more than cul-de-sacs off the information highway, to have them become a revolution in new tools to develop health-supporting communities.

Community Information Technology

Populations and Organizations

Each program targeted specific populations—patients and home caregivers, disadvantaged families, elders, teleworkers, city residents, and/or organizations: health and welfare agencies, local businesses, community organizations. They all offered information relevant to their targeted groups: databases on illness, commercial data, costs and services data, directories of available community services, and bulletin board announcements. Communication services included public forums and private electronic mail messaging and question-answer sessions with expert moderators. In addition, as in Southcity, organizations were supported by customized reports on their work and interaction aimed at coalition-building, and Westsun's public information network (PIN) allowed community mobilization around local issues. All systems were attempting to develop further services and none yet offered all that were possible and useful.

IT Support Services

The use of community IT depended on the support services that were available, beyond on-line and printed help. For individuals in Indy's CareNet, a team member called monthly and was on call for telephone or e-mail troubleshooting in addition to the initial personalized in-home set-up and training session. There were classroom training, tutoring, and supervised practice at Friends House's Computer Learning Center, as well as on-site set-up and staff training at nursing homes. On-site support was a service of the Southcity's Church Help Center and Westsun's city hall, which also had loanable videos for instruction and designated, trained IT coordinators at its public sites.

Outreach and Promotion

The capacity of each IT program for reaching its target group depended on its resources. These ranged from the Church Help Center's direct meetings with prospective user organizations to government access cable television by the city hall in Westsun. Most programs became known by the publicity generated through news and feature stories in local and wire press media; some were fortuitous, as in Southcity and Midcity, some carefully planned, as in Westsun.

Costs

The costs of community IT varied vastly, depending on the size and support of the parent organization. The essentials included pre-start-up staffing and funds, contacts and leverage with IT suppliers, technical assistance, and in-kind services like volunteer time and office space. The range in new monies used for the first year was fewer than $20,000 at Friends House to well over a million dollars for CareNet, a large share of which was for evaluation. The English Telecottage Association estimated that a teleservice center could begin with about $25,000 to $30,000 in the early 1990s.

Hardware

In almost every case, except for the relatively affluent Westsun city hall, matching low-cost components of the hardware—computers, printers, modems, telephone wiring—proved to be a problem, especially in linking older housing and facilities in disadvantaged communities. Rewiring and added telephone lines were too costly; potluck equipment made training trainers and support services more difficult.

Software

In every case, software was not suitable for the kinds of people-responsive services that community IT was intended to provide. The expert staff in Westsun programmed its system, but it took almost a year to do so. Indy had access to technical assistance as well as its own teams to develop its software as did Hill Park's Telebusiness Center. But the St. Francis Mobile Health Service had to design its own in collaboration with a software firm. And both Friends House and the Church Help Center were forced to hire programmers who turned out to have hidden proprietary agendas. Each site then had to seek additional help to repair the damage and redevelop their software.

Educational and other types of shareware, as a form of very low cost or free software, helped the low-budget programs. But for the Church Help Center's CHEC system, finding a way to develop an interagency database that included client data and information sharing while preserving both legal and ethical privacy rights remained a problem. This was as much a problem of agency politics as a technical and cost problem, and it illustrates the other essential for success in IT: the *soft* technology of organizational cooperation, the loosening of turf guarding, and collaborative resource development.

Parent Organizations

Environment

Each parent organization of community IT operated in an environment that supported community uses of IT, uses that went beyond conventional administrative and marketplace applications. Local electronic free-nets, school board IT programs, state incentives for "workstyle" changes, and funds from federal community development block grants, indicated a measure of public support and social acceptance for testing IT as a new set of tools to help address health, welfare, education, governance, and quality of life issues. In the eighties and early nineties, policy support in the United States was fragmented, tenuous, and difficult to find and use. In the United Kingdom and Europe, there were systematic, national policies to promote and support local IT development.

Impetus and Interests

The parent organizations in each case determined generally that "things are not as they should be" or could be, that their resources were not matching their mission adequately. That meant serving the community health needs of home caregivers, providing emergency aid to the homeless, offering enriching programs to neighborhood children and elders, creating jobs, or improving government responsiveness.

Alongside these service program problems were equally important strategic issues centering on the parent group's imperative to satisfy its constituencies, a major requisite to its survival. Generally, organizations must not only show that they are meeting their goals, but must do so in a manner that their sponsors, funders, donors, collaborators, and **potential** supporters approve (Hord 1986; Alter and Hage 1992). This meant that Indy College of Nursing's CareNet would give the college a community-responsive image to position it as a player in local health system reform, and a model for information age nursing. St. Francis's mobile IT in Southcity would attract funds that would pay for otherwise uncompensated care to the poor; the Computer Learning Center at Friends House would both please mainline congregations as a resource to do good and would attract support from neighborhood churches. Hill Park's Telebusiness Center was a form of job development that brought large funds from BT and from government sources, and the PIN network of Westsun's city hall got taxpayers' and voters' approval while maintaining the city's image of high-tech democratic governance, pleasing bureaucrats, councilors, and IT suppliers.

Enabling Contexts

The organizations that gave birth to community information technology became contexts for usable, mission-supporting IT innovations for nursing services, health and welfare for the homeless, nonformal education, economic development, and citizen participation. In some, like the college of nursing, a supportive structure was explicitly set up, with staff, discretionary funds, faculty time, and brokering to help shape community IT ideas. In others, the idea of community IT was brought into a ready setting by someone who agreed that "things are not as they should be" and was ready to try IT to help remedy the problems, as in Southcity's church council and Midcity's Friends House. St. Francis Health System, with its growing problem of financing care for the poor, scanned its programs, discovered the potential for new funds in the volunteer, mobile, IT-supported health service, and provided corporate backup to enable its success in grant-getting and expansion. The Hill Park Planning Board created an external enabling system, an endowed trust to fund action programs for the economic and social deficits in its region.

Leadership

In each case, there was a fit between the readiness of a parent organization that recognized its priority problems and an idea or vision bearer—"idea champion" (Galbraith 1982). The champion became a kind of CPU, to use a computer analogy, recruited by the organization as a willing agent to carry the idea, community IT, to fruition. The bearer seemed to be an individual, although in Westsun's city hall, it was the combination of a councilor, the Information Systems Department head, and his liberal university colleagues. The important condition for initiating the IT program was the mesh between the parent organization and a node of leadership that it would support to carry the innovation forward, not a lone, resourceless individual.

Organizing for Action

A variety of organizing units were devised by parent entities to develop community IT. Indy's College of Nursing used a multidisciplinary team with research and practitioner skills in health, social, and computer sciences and sought demonstration funds from foundations and evaluation funds from research institutes. Organizational coalitions were formed in Southcity knowing that federal funding would give priority to communities that could show they were working together. Friends House used its customary way of discovering new sources of funds—by being represented on many community boards—and its usual way of expanding its services—volunteers. In very different circumstances, Westsun's city hall used its Information Systems Department, which got new technology from the city's customary supplier network. The Hill Park Planning Board established a business-backed endowment trust to demonstrate its commitment to the community and then accepted a business-backed offer to use IT for economic development through paid staff and subcontractors.

The Development Process

Shaping the Idea

The initial community IT idea, computer services connected to homes, laptops, mainframes, support centers, and public sites, was not its final shape. Whom it would serve, how, and how long it would do so had to be molded to the interests of those who supplied the funds, technology, and expertise.

This constraint sometimes posed problems for the types of people that could be served. Indy's team developed an AIDS project because newly increased funds were available for that high-profile disease rather than using CareNet for mothers of premature babies. But funder interests expanded the range of beneficiaries when some of Southcity's fundamentalist and Catholic sponsors, as a condition for receiving certain public funds, allowed the CHEC and mobile IT programs to encompass AIDS groups and supply condoms and birth control information. Donor offers sometimes restricted the focus of the program, producing the profit-making aims of the Telebusiness Center at the behest of British Telecom for example. But donor netware encouraged expansion to Westsun's citizens when voters sought access to the electronic network that was initially available only to city hall officials.

Community IT programs were shaped too by the specific hardware and software available. This often meant dealing with incompatible equipment and software that could not be used on the available hardware. At the Friends Computer Learning Center, this made training trainers and teaching students difficult. It also meant, in Southcity, that some small churches could not join the CHEC network because old wiring and new telephone lines were beyond their budgets, as was true for some people living with AIDS in Indy.

Finding Resources

Progress required continuous efforts to address a number of problems simultaneously—to devise strategies that would move community IT through economic, political, and bureaucratic thickets to find sufficient resources. At the same time, the parent unit had to maneuver in ways to build its image among its constituents and supporters.

In the search for resources, the IT leaders first went through their familiar web of supporters, professional groups, or church or business associates. They then extended their reach to new potential parties, foundations, governments, and national firms. Part of negotiating skill was knowing where to search, to recognize a likely target, and to gather enough strategic information to be persuasive in showing how community IT would benefit the target organization (Zald and Useem 1987; Black 1983).

Negotiating the Essentials

The next best asset to having resources is the ability to convince those who have them to invest their wealth in a joint venture (Yutchman and Seashore 1967). Although certain intangible assets such as legitimacy, credibility, and reliability are often crucial to organizational survival, they rest on organizations' more readily measured resources of tangible wealth. Both types of assets are closely linked. Having hard assets usually confers an image of effectiveness, which in turn makes bargaining easier. Organized groups that are small, new, minimally resourced, and "different" in their aims have problems starting up and surviving (Minkoff 1993).

So it was with most of the incipient community IT programs in these cases. They used their parent organizations' strategic memories and organizational nets, and trial and error, though sometimes at high costs in time and energy. Negotiations had to address organizational interests and ensure enough cooperation for collaboration and coordination. But they found effective ways to get resource suppliers to commit enough funds, clients, technology, expertise, and facilities and staff to implement community IT.

Central to this bargaining was identifying the targeted source's potential gains and losses and then showing how the IT program would bring it a net gain. Obviously, community IT developed successfully in the cases cited because its sponsors won more bargaining encounters than they lost. How they gained the resources they needed illustrates both the difficulties and the types of accommodation that made community IT possible.

IT programs developed most easily, with fewer deadend bargaining episodes and reasonable assurance of survival, when they were attached to large or stable, longtime service organizations that were widely and well-connected in the community: PIN in Westsun's city hall; CareNet at Indy's college of nursing; St. Francis Mobile Health, and even the Computer Learning Center in Friends House. But both the Church Help Center in Southcity, which was poor, small, and freestanding, and the large, endowed Hill Park Trust were new and independent parent organizations and had to concern themselves with their own viability as well as tending to their IT offspring.

Although support from a strong parent group was an advantage, developers of community IT still had to convince targeted stakeholders to collaborate. CareNet showed nursing research funders that it would strengthen the traditional home support role of nurses in the information age. It convinced doctors that they would not lose control over their AIDS patients, the Alzheimer's Association chapter that it would gain clients as well as new software and hardware, and the Alzheimer's Center that its approach to information would be strengthened by testing CareNet and help its grant-getting efforts. All would benefit from favorable publicity with their respective publics, perhaps repositioning themselves a notch higher in their future bargaining.

The other sites used similar low or no cost-gains arguments, including intangible values, in their negotiations. After losing its encounter with the major players on its parent Council of Churches, which set absolute restrictions on the CHEC network, the Church Help Center had to emphasize intangible resources in its renewed search for funds. It showed social service organizations that CHEC could readily organize and interconnect services for all types of emergency aid clients and that there were many who were not being served. This appealed to funders who wanted proof that more money was needed to serve growing needs, and to very small service groups who believed that cooperation would help their own resource-getting efforts. Developing a track record, an image of service, would be helpful to all, including the IT manufacturers and retailers who provided discounted or free equipment.

Modeling

The modeling of community IT was itself a persuasive argument in many negotiations, as when the Church Help Center could show what CHEC had done; when the Hill Park Trust and BT could see what the Swedes had done; when CareNet could show the local Alzheimer's group's social workers that it would not make them obsolete; when the PIN pilot study became the rationale for citywide expansion in Westsun.

Accommodating Conflict

But successful negotiations at the outset did not guarantee smooth relations among collaborators, such as the CHEC network. There, partly because of the technical limits of the low-budget IT system, there were sometimes greater gains for some participating groups by leaving the system and developing their own network after they had gained the experience and seen the value of CHEC. The professional rivalries in the CareNet project required a mediating strategy to find a modestly satisfactory compromise. What finally cemented a workable relationship were the facts that each side could not reach its goals as a solo player and that their parent organizations wanted a workable relationship to be established. Both factors have been found to be important in other semicompetitive organizational pairs (Schermerhorn 1975; Gray 1989).

Yet, when two IT groups like Friends House and the SeniorNet program saw shared interests in close collaboration, both gaining in clients, staff, and program services, they were able to maintain a mutually beneficial relationship. As in similar cooperative relations, their previous successful experiences and willingness to share credit, recognizing their mutual needs and interdependence, augured well for future joint efforts (Hord 1986; Schermerhorn 1975; Perrow 1993).

In Westsun, elected officials found ways to tolerate the sometimes blatant namecalling on PIN as part of the larger benefits of the city's image as a high-tech democracy and the growing perception that public networks would be cost-saving utilities that governments would have to offer a computer literate citizenry.

All types of organizations have interests at stake as they interact with each other, whether they are governmental, commercial, scientific, medical, or voluntary, nonprofit groups (Feldstein 1988; Bergthold 1990; Austin and Overholt 1988; Warner 1991; DiMaggio and Anheier 1990). The community cases illustrate how success in getting and holding essential resources for development and operation of community IT depended on negotiating relationships with potential stakeholders by persuading them that any stake in the venture would do them little harm and enough good to make their expenditure worthwhile. Any signs of conflict arising from changing circumstances in the organizations and their environments had to be constantly monitored and resolved to maintain enough cooperation to allow collaboration to continue.

Using Information in Community IT Development

What place did information have in the development of community information technology? In the most basic terms, people use only two currencies in their interchanges: information and physical force. Excluding physical force, all other forms of negotiation, ranging from enticement to intimidation and threat of force, require information to convey the message. Even when the incentive is money or other forms of wealth, convincing information about its availability is necessary.

So progress in community IT negotiations meant that its bearers were able develop and use the right information at the right time with the right stakeholders. It meant they learned what their prospective partners' interests were and framed their proposals in ways that took those interests into account. They developed strategic information ("intelligence") and used information to serve strategic ends, to move community IT from an idea to a sustainable reality.

Types of Information

The development of community IT, like most program development, required three basic types of information: technical (hard data, such as that to ensure IT system quality); managerial or organizational (on how to put all the resources together to function effectively); and strategic (the requisite for effective bargaining). Arguably, strategic information was most important, if only because it preceded the other forms in order to obtain the expertise and other resources for the projects.

The IT parent organizations, for example, scanned their group environments to find the sources they could target for funds. When they used factual data or scientifically acquired information, they used it strategically, to persuade stakeholders. But "facts" always remained a minor component in negotiations, as when the Hill Park Trust determined its choice for an economic development strategy before the regional study it had commissioned was completed. If technical data were of primary importance, the hard-line stance of some of Southcity's churches would have been softened when factual information on the needs of the homeless were presented to them. Some of them were persuaded to alter their positions only when they obtained other (strategic) information—namely, the availability of federal funds for providing AIDS, birth control, and other services. The pilot test of PIN in Westsun was known to be a way to justify (for strategic ends) what was already an unofficial political decision, rather than a scientific experiment to determine whether PIN was feasible and effective.

Science and verifiable, hard information has rarely been decisive or even persuasive in organizational negotiations about program or policy development (Brint 1990). Although hard information is often used, the purpose is almost always strategic: to justify choices that are determined on a political, negotiated basis, on trade-offs between the major stakeholders in a particular situation (Laumann and Knoke 1987).

The Impact of Community Information Technology

Individuals

The general public and the specific publics that each variant of community IT focused on were able to obtain an array of information, to become computer literate, and in some settings, to get basic services such as medical and nursing advice, translation services, library books, and referral services. But as the CareNet evaluation showed, the most popular services on the network were group and individual communication. The most rational use, the decision support module, was the one least used. Perhaps it was best said by the right-wing leader in Westsun, "People do not crave new sources of information so much as new venues for talking to one another."

In both Indy and Westsun, where surveys were done, there passive readers outnumbered the active scribes by perhaps 3 to 1. The readers were participants, nonetheless, viewing the on-screen discussions on themes of their own choosing and stimulating, reinforcing, or challenging their own views on selected issues. In Westsun, these audiences included city policymakers who chose not to expose themselves to open dialog on the network.

Organizations

A still less expected result of people talking electronically was that they wanted to meet face-to-face—even the Alzheimer's caregivers who had severe constraints on leaving home. Users also formed "virtual"—electronic—and formal, incorporated organizations capable of taking actions that made a difference in their communities. These groups included, perhaps more so than conventionally organized groups, a wider diversity of members who could join in on-line as they wished, revealing as much or as little about themselves as they wanted.

So community IT became more than a way to deliver health, social, educational, and business information and services, and more than a means for the parent organizations and participating groups to develop new services and extend their programs at relatively little cost. Community IT also became a vehicle for organization and advocacy. In a sense it was a medium for growing new organizations and renewing old ones.

References

Alter, C., and J. Hage. 1992. *Organizations Working Together: Coordination in Interorganizational Networks*. Newbury Park: Sage Publications.

Austin, J., and C. Overholt. 1988. "Nutrition Policy: Building the Bridge between Science and Politics." *Annual Review of Nutrition* 8: 1–20.

Bergthold, L. 1990. *Purchasing Power in Health, Business, the State, and Health Care Politics*. New Brunswick, NJ: Rutgers University Press.

Black, T. R. 1983. "Coalition Building—Some Suggestions." *Child Welfare* 62 (May/June): 263–68.

Brint, S. 1990. "Rethinking the Policy Influence of Experts: From General Characterizations to Analysis of Variation." *Sociological Forum* 5 (3): 361–85.

DiMaggio, P., and H. Anheier. 1990. "The Sociology of Non-Profit Organizations and Sectors." *Annual Review of Sociology* 16: 137–59.

Feldstein, P. J. 1988. *The Politics of Health Legislation. An Economic Perspective*. Ann Arbor, MI: Health Administration Press.

Galbraith, J. 1982. "Designing the Innovating Organization." *Organization Dynamics* (Winter): 5–25.

Gray, B. 1989. *Collaborating: Finding Common Ground for Multiparty Problems*. San Francisco: Jossey-Bass.

Hord, S. M. 1986. "A Synthesis of Research on Organizational Collaboration." *Educational Leadership* (February): 22–26.

Laumann, E., and D. Knoke. 1987. *The Organizational State*. Madison, WI: University of Wisconsin Press.

Minkoff, D. 1993. "The Organization of Survival: Women's and Racial-Ethnic Voluntarist and Activist Organizations, 1955–1985." *Social Forces* 71 (June): 887–908.

Perrow, C. 1993. "Organizational Theorists in a Society of Organizations." *International Society* 7 (September): 371–80.

Schermerhorn, J. R. 1975. "Determinants of Interorganizational Cooperation." *Academy of Management Journal* 18 (December): 846–56.

Warner, K. 1991. "Tobacco Industry Scientific Advisors: Serving Society or Selling Cigarettes?" *American Journal of Public Health* 81 (7): 839–42.

Yuchtman, E., and S. Seashore. 1967. "A System Resource Approach to Organizational Effectiveness." *American Sociological Review* 32: 891–903.

Zald, M., and B. Useem. 1987. "Movement and Countermovement Interactions: Mobilization, Tactics, and State Involvement." *Social Movements in an Organizational Society* (Special Issue): 247–72.

PART

III

POLICYMAKING

. . . We will not live in a true information society unless—and until—we ensure that people have affordable public access to government information. We will not live in a true information society unless—and until—people have the skills and resources to use this information. We will not live in a true information society unless—and until—public policy makers recognize that an informed citizenry is a public good that benefits us all. . . .

American Library Association, 1992

The new technologies hold promise for a greatly enhanced system that can meet the changing needs of an information-based society. At the same time, these technologies will generate a number of significant social problems. How these technologies evolve, as well as who will be affected positively or negatively, will depend on decisions now being made in both the public and private sectors. . . . making choices about universal service is essentially making choices about equality of opportunity. Defining universal service is, in effect, making choices about the nature of society itself.

Office of Technology Assessment,
U.S. Congress, *Critical Connections*, 1990

INTRODUCTION TO PART III

THIS SECTION focuses on the information technology policy environment and issues that policymakers chose to address in the early and mid-1990s. It also points to issues they did not address. The consequences of both action and inaction for the future of disadvantaged communities relate to whether they will be provided with the information technology tools to build health-supporting institutions and environments, or whether they will be bypassed and fall further behind their more advantaged counterparts.

In Chapter 15 the policy world is pictured in the light of past information and communications policies, proposed legislative and regulatory changes, and the players involved in the decision-making actions. The point is made that even public interest groups, attempting to speak for the public good, conceived the public interest in individual terms, not giving much attention to the problems faced by low-income communities.

The final chapter, Chapter 16, provides some observations derived from my participation in a few of the forums shaping the national information infrastructure since my initial inquiry and offers some recommendations for information technology policy to develop information technology capacity in disadvantaged communities and organizations as a means to build healthy communities.

CHAPTER

15

THE INFORMATION TECHNOLOGY POLICY ENVIRONMENT

WIDESPREAD RECOGNITION that technological possibility could soon become social reality emerged in the 1990s. The vision of a national information infrastructure—the "seamless web" of communications networks encompassing broadcast, cable, telephone wire, optical fiber, satellite, microwave, and information media (TV, computers, compact discs, and video)—was crystallized and given a high profile with the election of a new federal administration in 1992. It was later endorsed by the leadership of both political parties.

Within a month of taking office, the Clinton-Gore administration announced a Technology Initiative as its strategy for economic development and job creation:

> American technology must move in a new direction. . . . Our most important measure of success will be our ability to make a difference in the lives of the American people, to harness technology so that it improves the quality of their lives and the economic strength of our nation. . . . We are moving to accelerate the development of civilian technology with new criteria. . . . Improving the skills offered by American workers by increasing the productivity and the accessibility of education and training. . . . Supporting communities or disadvantaged groups . . . who have not enjoyed the benefits of technology-based economic growth. . . . (Clinton and Gore 1993, 1, 3)

Six months later the Administration laid out "An Agenda for Action" for accelerating the development of the NII, promising to commit $1 billion to $2 billion a year to support the development of telecommunications and information infrastructure through expanded research and development, demonstration and testing, education and training, standard setting and quality control, as well as regulatory changes to encourage industry investment beyond the annual $50 billion already being spent (NTIA 1993). Estimates of the costs of the NII over 10 to 15 years were $400 billion based on full installation of optical fiber networks, although the use of newer wireless technologies or the use of older unused parts of the radio spectrum lowered that estimate considerably (Newman et al. 1993; Sirbu 1992).

The agenda also aimed to extend access at affordable prices to all Americans, especially those in disadvantaged and rural communities. The intention was to improve access to government information and enhance government efficiency through information technology. These directions were further spelled out in the vice president's "Report on the National Performance Review of the Federal Government." It envisioned providing food stamp benefits electronically, integrating federal IT systems, ensuring privacy and security of data, and training federal employees to use IT networks (Gore 1993). Some public interest groups were wary of some of these proposals. Digitized food stamp payments, for example, would track food purchases of low-income people, monitoring to which others were not subjected, and could also allow their records to be linked to national electronic police databases, again an intrusion not asked of or likely to be tolerated by others.

The Political Arena

The NII vision gave strong impetus to an already active policy arena and drew in old and new stakeholder groups that sought a place at the negotiating table as the goals—which all agreed were laudable—were determined by policies. The field of contention and compromise was populated by industry associations, public interest groups, educational and research institutions, think tanks and foundations, and religious and consumer groups, along with federal, state, and local government agencies, and congressional committees. All sought to protect and enhance their interests as the NII took shape. At stake were economic and ideological interests, political bargaining power, and bureaucratic and budgetary control as each group or set of allies attempted to get its particular vision of NII ensured and enshrined in public policy.

Dissolving Old Media

The older information media—newspapers and magazines—had a 200-year history of almost no regulation through the First Amendment freedoms to speak, hear, and know, as fundamental to a democratic society. Radio and TV have been licensed since the early thirties to serve "the public interest, convenience and necessity" (McChesney 1993). In return for the use of the publicly owned and finite broadcast spectrum, sections of which are reserved for noncommercial use, they were held to "equal-time" rules (requiring the lowest unit charge for advertising by all political candidates) and the "fairness" doctrine. License holders had to offer "discussions of controversial issues" and "expression of opposing views" enforced by the Federal Communications Commission. This doctrine, as well as the requirement to "ascertain and serve local community needs" and provide news, public affairs and children's programming, was changed to a mere admonition in the deregulatory climate of the 1980s. "Cross-ownership" among mass media in a single media market was also loosened, allowing multimedia ownership (Love 1993b).

Cable, developing in the seventies, was never subject to programming content rules because of the technical possibility of very large numbers of transmission channels in contrast to the restricted radio spectrum. Local franchising authorities could, however, require systems to provide public, educational, and government (PEG) access channels and production facilities for locally produced programming.

Telephone companies, in return for the monopoly privileges they had for local telephone service, operated as "common carriers." They could not refuse to sell services to any information-provider companies.

Regulatory Mismatch

Emerging telecommunication and information technologies and their foreseeable electronic merger as a national information infrastructure are producing rule changes through the courts and legislation, and require a reexamination of the regulatory system that was based on separable and independent media. Cellular phones and personal communication services (PCS)—wireless pocket devices combining telephone, portable computer, and fax capabilities—are competing with local telephone services; newpapers are supplying information on-line through computers and cable systems; computers allow televised entertainment through compact discs.

Court rulings in the nineties determined that phone companies could not be barred under the First Amendment from offering information services, such as newspaper articles and databases, or "video dial tone" services, such as cable pay-per-view movies. Nor could they be stopped from entering joint ventures or mergers with companies producing these services, including cable companies ("Calling" 1993).

These mushrooming technological and commercial realities merged "content and conduit," the capacity of large corporations to be the gatekeepers of information content and of the transmission conduits to users worldwide. These multibillion-dollar firms would very likely become few in number and not very competitive because there could be few sources of large-scale alternative financing outside the entertainment industry.

A new, looser regulatory framework, while meeting the administration's goal of freeing industry to accelerate investment in infrastructure and new services, would also have to address ways to ensure affordable access to diverse sources of information through a true competitive market. In the view of public interest groups, it ought to reserve some public space in the infrastructure for noncommercial and free use, modeled after the existing Internet.

Internet

The Internet digital computer network was developed in the late 1960s as ARPANET and was funded by the Pentagon's Advanced Research Projects Agency (ARPA). Smaller, separate networks were set up for university and commercial purposes in the next decade when the electronic bulletin board system was begun and the first public terminal was set up in Berkeley, California. During the 1980s, the National Science Foundation devised NSFnet for five university-based research centers. The first community political action bulletin board was also set up in Colorado, the first course for college credit was taught entirely on-line, and the first citywide freenet began in Cleveland (Morino Institute 1994).

All the while, software was being designed to interconnect these networks to arrive at the Internet of the nineties. The Internet now interconnects over 11,000 networks in over 100 countries with over 37 million users in universities, governments, libraries, and businesses worldwide, about 17 million of them in the United States. Three to five million Americans use paid subscriber services on private and commercial networks (Smarr and Catlett 1992).

By the early 1990s, most universities and community colleges were part of the Internet and about 1,000 high schools had joined. With legislation introduced by then-Senator Al Gore, Internet, now the largest computer network in the world, was to be upgraded to become the National Research and Educational Network (NREN)—allowing all education and research institutions to join. Internet has been coordinated and continuously improved by the Internet Activities Board as an entirely voluntary, nonprofit, cooperative system, with a rapidly growing for-profit subsidiary for commercial IT service providers. Anyone with computer, modem, and password could use its vast menu of free or commercial services (Cooke and Lehrer 1993; Newman et al. 1993).

Shaping Policy for the Information Highway

The Major Issues

As the merging of new information technologies makes clear, there are unimagined possibilities for new kinds of public and commercial activity, both organized and individual. In the past, federal law and regulation pursued separate tracks in dealing with the conduits and the content of information media, regulating each in sometimes different ways, as noted. The efforts to reconceive the new worlds that were made possible by technologies and developed in large part with public funds drew in every affected group.

The major issues of contention over the next several years concerned control of the NII: whether and to what extent it should be dominated by the large telecommunications-information industry conglomerates. In other words, what was to be the meaning of "universal service," how should it be financed, and who should decide? There was broad agreement on allowing limited free "testbed" uses for experimenting with innovations and education, granting special status to scientists, educators, and students. But this arrangement would call into question the meaning of universal access, which involved costs to the user, access sites, equipment for accessing the NII, and training and ongoing support for users. Regardless of the *extent* of access, another set of issues involved the *kinds* and *number* of IT services—information, communication, video, voice, graphics, and data—to be available to the ordinary user.

Public opinion polls suggested that large majorities of voters favored an active government role in addressing access and cost issues. Three-quarters said that government should provide grants to help communities make the new technologies available in nonprofit groups, schools, libraries, and hospitals. Similar numbers thought that companies that profited from the new technologies should be required to commit a part of their resources to support community uses and community access to government information. Two-thirds of voters believed that government should support technology-delivered adult education courses to home, ensure access to everyone, and provide information to teach people how to use IT (Lake 1994).

The interested parties lined up on various sides of the issues of universality, financing, regulation, and control.

The Players

Industry

A month after the announcement of the Technology Initiative, the nation's 14 largest telecommunications firms issued a joint policy statement laying out their position on the role that government should play in developing the NII. They wanted private industry to build and operate the NII and have government share the cost. They wanted government to buy (rather than develop) services for use on the NII, even those on the testbed, which itself would be financed by public funds. Public funds would also develop the IT capacity, network connections, user-friendly software, and subsidized use of commercial services for local governments, libraries, schools, and health facilities. The industry sought to prevent having the Internet named in legislation or other policy statements, claiming this would be anticompetitive with commercially available networks. Finally, the group wanted to implement the transition to the NII with government, and to have official representation from the computer, telecommunications, information, and related industries in the decision-making processes (Subcommittee on Science 1993).

The Computer Systems Policy Project funded by the country's 13 largest computer companies, also espoused a "true partnership" between industry and government. Public funds would finance basic research and demonstration projects, and federal leadership would shape the vision of NII that the private sector would build and manage. It foresaw, for example, the NII improving the delivery of health care through better information management, insurance claims processing, and medical access to databases and to expert clinicians through telemedicine. Self-care information would be sent to individuals in their homes. Government would make its information easily accessible to the public using industry hardware and software, ensure "a level playing field for all technologies," and adopt interoperability standards developed by industry. Finally, government would catalyze, cajole, and coordinate public-private resolution of such issues as access; free expression of ideas on NII, privacy, security, and confidentiality; affordability; protection of intellectual property; and regulatory barriers to new technologies (Subcommittee on Science 1993).

The Computer and Communications Industry Association urged the government not to "reinvent the wheel," which the private technology market had in hand, and cautioned that it was "important not to keep *anybody* from accessing NII services just because *everybody* can't have it." Tolerance of IT haves and have-nots, in other words, was a satisfactory policy to adopt (OMB 1993b).

The Information Industry Association (IIA), representing 500 global and domestic companies in publishing, database production and delivery, interactive electronic services, and software developers, emphasized the commercial value of information. While it did not advocate that government should be banned from providing information that the private sector could provide, it wanted a competitive marketplace in information services "clearly stated in the law," as well as representation on policy advisory committees. Government "should steer and not row." The industry pointed to its own key role in value-added production, such as adding indexing and other aids to government information, providing multiple distribution channels, and giving ongoing customer support. The IIA wanted government agencies to be mandated to assess the competitive impact on the private sector before they decided to disseminate public information through IT. It also wanted state and local governments forbidden from asserting copyright for public information provided in federally funded NII demonstrations (Subcommittee on Science 1993; OMB 1993b).

The Cellular Communications Industry Association wanted more emphasis in research and development placed on wireless technologies, such as personal communications, satellite networks, and cellular telephones, which are now available to more than 60 percent of the public, rather than predominantly wireline technologies, such as fiber optics (OTA 1993b).

A Public Commercial Alliance

The Coalition for Networked Information, begun in 1990 as the first legislation on networking was introduced, combined the interests of scholars, researchers, and teachers in higher education and the commercial interests of publishers and IT hardware and software companies. The group wanted to ensure its inclusion at the table so that the government would not "duplicate" or "overlook" its experience and expertise. It also was studying ways to commercialize NREN (Committee on Rules 1992).

The Education Sector

Somewhat in contrast, the Institute for Academic Technology, made up of universities and colleges, wanted guarantees that all federal information would be available electronically to citizens in convenient, friendly formats without cost, and that the 1,400 federal depository libraries, on which universities rely, would have an important role in this information and technology transfer mission (Committee on Rules 1992).

A group representing primarily midwestern, public systems, the National Association of State Universities and Land-Grant Colleges, was concerned that access and affordability of information on NREN be ensured. It also pointed out the advantage of having a support system, MIDNET, a kind of mediating organization, to assist its member groups in developing and using IT. MIDNET, serving seven states, negotiated with networking firms to provide their services to campuses; purchased and installed the equipment needed to connect to the Internet and the software for new applications; and monitored and supported the network and its users, as well as trained trainers for the campuses and assisted them in collaborative work. The need for an ongoing support system was clear, even for the sophisticated information and technology users in American higher education (Subcommittee on Science 1993).

Congressional Interests

The views from the House Select Subcommittee on Education and Civil Rights, the only voice of its kind in the NII Hearings of 1993, pointed to the federal role and responsibility in eliminating the distinction between the "information poor" and "information rich" in underserved urban and rural areas. The committee was especially concerned about access for the disabled. NII should expand equality of opportunity, promoting full participation for all. A "universally accessible network" should not cost the disabled more than others, even though special equipment would be needed by those with limited sensory or movement capacity (Subcommittee on Science 1993).

An array of authorizing committees in both the House and the Senate dealt with information and telecommunications policies. Action focused on the information policies committees in the first session and on the telecommunications committees in the last half of the 103rd Congress in 1994. The most active were the House Committee on Administration Subcommittee on Government Affairs, Committee on Science, Space, and Technology; Committee on Education and Labor Subcommittee on Elementary, Secondary, and Vocational Education; the Agricultural Subcommittees on Rural Development and Operations, and the Subcommittee on Telecommunications of the Committee on Energy and Commerce. Senate counterparts included the Rules Subcommittee on Government Operations, the Labor and Human Resources Committee, and the Committee on Commerce, Science, and Transportation Subcommittee on Communications. Each committee had its own constituencies and its own priority issues commensurate with its jurisdiction and supporters, and so was itself a contender in the political give-and-take.

Public Interest Groups

The fervent activity shaping the NII in the 1990s recalled an earlier revolution in information and communication at the birth of American broadcasting in the late twenties and thirties. Then as now there was contention between those who saw the new technology as a private and profit-making industry and others who saw it as a free public service under public control.

The public interest reformers from civic groups, churches, education, and other nonprofit organizations lost the debate six decades ago. They could not convince their own members that broadcasting was a crucial development, nor could they rally consistent public support. Compared with their corporate adversaries, they had meager resources. Their coalition split into rival groups when some sided with the broadcasters as representatives of free speech who promised to freely donate time for public interest issues. Commercial groups held up to Congress the vision of a private system that would create jobs and tax revenues—a system having little controversy and needing little governmental oversight. Finally, the broadcasters simply neglected to cover the issues over the airwaves—similar to the last decade, which has seen little exposure in the mass media of the issues, interests, alternatives, and potential consequences of the NII, apart from mega-deals and consumer products (McChesney 1993).

A New Coalition

Today's merging of computer, telephone, and television technologies into national interconnected digital networks, and the merging of public policies to enable and regulate them, also moved public interest organizations to come together as the Telecommunications Policy Roundtable in 1993. The more than 50 groups were first convened by OMB Watch, a ten-year-old independent watchdog over the Office of Management and Budget, the agency that directs the release of government information. They agreed on a set of principles for the design of the NII, and were represented by libraries, teachers, consumers, voters, writers, artists, community broadcasters, public television stations, historians, sports fans, the disabled, and civil liberties and participatory democracy advocates. These groups included Public Citizen, Taxpayer Assets Project, the Center for Media Education, Center for Civic Networking, American Library Association, and Computer Professionals for Social Responsibility.

The aim was to ensure an "electronic commons" for the public, a public lane in the information superhighway, guaranteed by the federal government. Their seven principles included: universal access—meaning affordable news, public affairs, education, health, and government information and free access to services "essential to fully participate in a democratic society"; freedom to communicate, where two-way audio-video routes are open to every individual and group; a "vital civic sector," ensuring a way to build communities through free interchange among groups, a diverse and competitive marketplace, and the absolute division between carriers and content providers; and democratic policymaking in the development and ongoing regulation of the NII (Telecommunications Policy Roundtable 1993).

Organization Agendas

As with the commercial associations, each organization in the Roundtable also belonged to other coalitions and espoused more detailed positions of special importance to its own constituency. The Center for Media Education wanted to prevent the NII from becoming a "vast shopping mall," seeing this as detrimental to democracy. It emphasized antitrust enforcement and ensuring noncommercial programming and services, such as state and local counterparts of C-SPAN, multicultural programming, and independent producer initiatives. New sources of financing should include a nonprofit group rate structure comparable to nonprofit postal rates (Bollier 1993).

The Communications Act, which regulated the media since 1934, ought to be amended to enact a "new social contract" between the telecommunications industry and the American people, according to the Electronic Frontier Foundation, a nonprofit group that promoted civil liberties in the digital media. The architecture of the electronic superhighway should be designed to provide "open platform" services. Unlike today's channel-based cable TV system where program producers must contract with cable firms, an open platform network would allow every person to have direct access to the entire superhighway. This would mean that programmers—any individuals and small organizations who could interest consumers—could distribute information of every type directly to consumers, literally a free and open marketplace for ideas and commerce.

The terms of the social contract would require guarantees from the large companies controlling the networks that they would be "common carriers" (as are telephone companies), allowing all programmers access to their platform and that they would interconnect with all other networks seamlessly. Firms that sell entertainment or other services would keep their customers' buying records confidential and agree to legal guidelines for individual control over access to and reuse of personal user information. And costs to consumers would be affordable to ensure universal access. Where an open and competitive electronic market would inevitably exclude organizations with limited resources, such as schools, libraries, and small community groups, their access would be subsidized through, for example, federal funds or a tax on the companies that control the network.

Thus the foundation's position on the NII stood between those who opposed giant media mergers and those who advocated a completely competitive market to shape the information network. They held that Congress should make the mergers hinge on detailed commitments according to the tenets of a new legal framework recodified in the Communications Act (Kapor and Berman 1993).

OMB Watch viewed access to government information as a means for negotiating and influencing regulatory rule making, a way to build community responsiveness in government and industry, and a tool for "reinventing government" (Bass and MacLean 1993).

The Taxpayer Assets Project sought accountability of government departments in the provision of information and from commercial conduit and content providers, for adherence to a modernized version of the equal time and fairness doctrines (Love 1993a).

Computer Professionals for Social Responsibility wanted access to the NII from homes and from public terminals at libraries, schools, and other public places to be free to the user for government-related information, communication, and services, supported by staff assistance with public funds. It also sought government support for community networks, through training, subsidies, and user-friendly IT, and provision of local social, cultural, governmental, and educational services through local organizations (CPSR 1993, 1994).

The Center for Civic Networking saw the NII as a means to rebuild a sense of community among users and revitalize civic participation, strengthening local governmental, service, and cultural institutions (Civille, Fidelman, and Altobello 1993). Access to information would enable people to more easily address problems right in their own homes, for self-care, formal and nonformal education, emergency services, sustainable development, small business management, and job training and access to employment markets. It also pointed to the importance of using "benchmarks" to monitor whether the benefits for individuals were actually being achieved.

Other public interest advocates, such as the Institute for Policy Studies, emphasized the importance of rebuilding geographic communities through the uses of IT and enabling those most affected to participate in the process through IT (Institute for Policy Studies 1993). In a similar way, the Corporation for Public Broadcasting, which finances the public broadcasting network, supported communitywide education and information services (CWEIS) based on the NII as a way to strengthen and improve the general well-being of "communities of place," in the same way that shared public infrastructures like local telephone, transportation, and utility systems support and bind communities. This they contrasted with "communities of interest," which are bound by communication and information sharing but are widely dispersed (CPB 1993).

In more hands-on ways, the Center for Community Change, which supported 100 community development organizations across the country and linked them electronically through its CommunityLink network, pointed out the importance of having staff support to maintain services and train and retrain user groups because of rapid local staff turnover.

Without access to outside funds or lower support costs, the center held that NII would bypass low-budget local organizations.

A Public Interest Summit

Within a year of the first meeting of the Telecommunications Roundtable, public interest group activity resulted in a "Public Interest Summit" with the Vice-President. The event was hosted by the Benton Foundation because some groups objected to a government-sponsored site. It was an effort to get a hearing within the Clinton administration for the coalition's concerns to help offset what it saw as the far greater attention paid to industry interests. In essence, the coalition juxtaposed two futures for the NII. One "could improve health care, enrich education and life-long learning, foster an informed public active in its own governance, and drive a competitive economy supporting new, well-paid jobs." But without the participation of nonprofit groups in shaping the NII, the alternative would be a "national amusement infrastructure built for games, movies, and shopping" (Benton Foundation 1994a).

Legislation

Communications Policy

A few months later with concerted effort, some of it face-to-face and much of it over the Internet, the Public Right-of-Way Act was introduced in the Senate as an amendment to pending telecommunications legislation. The bill called for reserving up to 20 percent of the capacity of advanced telecommunications networks for use by state and local governments, educational institutions, public broadcasters, libraries, and nonprofit groups providing educational, informational, cultural, civic, and social welfare services. It also provided a funding mechanism to enable these groups to use the networks.

Other legislation suggested the outlines of the new NII (OMB 1993c). Extending access to Internet/NREN, funds were provided to connect public schools, libraries, governments, health care facilities, and other nonprofit institutions and to demonstrate how the NII interconnections could enhance the services of these local agencies. Twenty-six million dollars was appropriated in 1994 and $64 million was budgeted for fiscal 1995, much less than the Administration sought.

Other bills proposed to end the legal local telephone monopolies of the Regional Bell Operating Companies and allowed them to provide information services, including dial-up video dialtone for instant access to a potentially huge library of movies, billed to one's telephone account. The conditions placed on this expansion included, for both telephone and cable companies, allowing any new information service providers to interconnect with their communications lines (maintaining "common carrier" status and providing universal access to a set of basic public services with preferential rates for public and nonprofit groups). "Electronic redlining" (bypassing disadvantaged areas with low market potential) and "cross-subsidies" (shifting the new costs of new services to universal basic telephone and cable service rates) were prohibited (Benton Foundation 1994b). Although the meanings of universal public access and universal services varied among several bills, these concepts became key issues in the debate, whereas in the previous Congress they had been almost invisible.

Legislation also called for improving access to IT for underserved classrooms, development of a clearinghouse on technologies to assist distance learning program development, and support for establishing state-based electronic libraries.

Information Policy

These proposals addressed hardware and financing of the NII, the "conduits." Other bills dealt with content, the amount, quality, and security of the information to be publicly available through IT. The importance of these policies lies in the fact that the federal government is the largest single producer, collector, consumer, and disseminator of information in the country, and by implication, the world (OMB 1993a).

The Improvement of Information Access Act passed in 1993, for example, required federal agencies for the first time to use diverse modes of dissemination, especially through electronic technologies, to provide information to the federal depository libraries across the country, and to ensure free or lowest cost access to the public through the Internet. Using standard formats, offered in timely and reliable ways, the Government Printing Office, a prime source of public information, was to place online a directory of all available government information as well as the Congressional Record and the Federal Register, which holds all proposed regulations made available for public comment.

This legislation was in line with an executive order issued early in the Clinton administration that reversed the policy of the two previous administrations (Bass and Plocher 1989; Love 1993a). Instead of privatizing government information (allowing the private sector to supply it on a commercial basis), it asserted that government information was a "valuable national resource. . . . essential to a democratic society. . . . a means to ensure accountability. . . . manage government operations. . . . maintain healthy performance of the economy. . . ." as well as being a commodity in the marketplace. It directed all federal agencies to take the initiative in providing information to the public using electronic tools wherever feasible at least cost, and also to make it available to the Government Printing Office, which in principle could supply it free to the library system (OMB 1993a).

Although these kinds of government information may not be of immediate interest to the average individual, they are pertinent to the concerns of many small groups and organizations. With free and timely access to program and policy-relevant information, these groups could take action with the speed and accuracy that have usually been possible only for larger, well-funded groups with Washington-based connections.

Structures Defining the Vision and the Reality

The organized and competing interests of commercial and public interest groups, backed by unequal funds, staff, and technology, contended to have their voice and vision represented in the machinery set up by the NII Agenda for Action. The chief NII policymaking body was the Information Infrastructure Task Force, a group of high-level representatives of the federal agencies with a major role in the NII, chaired by the Secretary of Commerce. This was a distinct shift from previous years of locating the lead IT agency in the Defense Department. Funds for development of high-performance computing that were initially authorized for NASA and the Department of Energy were shifted to such agencies as the National Science Foundation and Health and Human Services to develop NII demonstration programs, all signaling a different emphasis in IT than previous administrations had taken (Committee on Science 1993).

The task force was to design a national strategy to promote the development of the NII, the "integration of hardware, software, and skills to make it easy and affordable to connect people with each other, with computers, and with a vast array of services and information resources" (White House 1993). The group was to point out what roles the public and private sectors would play to ensure maximum benefits for new jobs and productivity, quality of life, and democracy through "electronic commerce, agile manufacturing, life-long learning, health care, government services, and civic networking," and to ensure universal access and personal privacy. The public interest groups, who believed that their agenda and voice were excluded from the charge, took heart after noting that as a result of meetings with White House staff, "democracy" and "civic networking" were added to the charge. They were hopeful that one or two places on the Task Force advisory council would be held for their formal input.

The council was appointed to represent the views of public- and private-sector interests. The 30 members included representatives of the telecommunications and entertainment industries, education and labor, local and state governments, libraries, the disabled, and one public interest organization regarded as centrist in its policy stance (NTIA 1994).

Formally the NII Task Force was staffed by the National Telecommunications and Information Administration and obtained technical advice from the machinery set up under the White House Office of Science and Technology Policy to carry out previous high-performance computing and the national research and education network legislation. This also had an industry advisory group, but was later expanded by Congress to include education, consumer, and public interest representation (Committee on Science 1993).

The Task Force's working groups, chaired by government agency heads, focused on telecommunications, including universal access and NII applications and federally funded demonstrations, at about $90 million over two years, to show how local governments, schools, libraries, and health care services could use electronic networks to improve the efficiency and quality of services. The other focus was on how to provide access to government information. This group proposed the Government Information Locator Service (GILS) to help the public locate and access information throughout the federal government. It would be used directly from users' computers or through intermediaries like libraries, kiosks, fax machines, "800" numbers, compact discs, and print.

Every unit in this NII planning structure offered a formal channel for influencing decisions on the shape of the NII. It also afforded informal access to officials and others representatives of competing visions—if they could learn the correct route, reach their destination at timely moments, and especially if they could count on intermediaries to smooth the path.

The Congressional Maze

Another set of parties involved in the construction of the information highway, perhaps even more complex and disparate, were the committees of Congress that controlled the legislation and regulatory agencies on telecommunications and information, and the appropriations that could put a vision in place. Administrative committees in the Senate and House dealt with access to government information (in the House, information shares a subcommittee with justice and agriculture); science committees dealt with technologies; education and health committees dealt with applications of technologies; appropriations committees supplied funds;

and oversight committees examined the agencies responsible for carrying out the legislation. There remained little incentive to change this complex IT committee structure because changes could threaten hard-earned chairships and the resources, staff, and influence that accompany them.

Congress also had several outside bodies to help inform its decisions, all of which were involved in the issues facing NII policy. These include the Congressional Budget Office, which estimates costs; the Congressional Research Service, which develops background information; the Office of Technology Assessment, which projects future prospects and recommends options; and the General Accounting Office, which assesses the implementation of legislation.

Movement toward a Framework

Partly because IT changed so quickly in recent years, neither the congressional decision-making setup nor legislation kept pace. This allowed many points of access for outside input, but it also created a thicket in which both lobbyists and policymakers had to find coherence and consensus to guide the NII. At the same time, there were signs in the 103rd Congress that a concerted effort to develop coherence had begun.

There was promise in the Senate, as noted, of amending the regulatory framework of the Communications Act, and of rethinking the earlier High Performance Computer and Communications Act to place greater emphasis on IT applications in civilian life, renaming it the National Information Infrastructure Act of 1993 (Committee on Science 1993). Government information was reconceived as an important part of the NII due to the new public interest emphasis of information policy issued under the executive order through OMB, and enacted as the Improvement of Information Access Act (Love 1992; Committee on House Administration 1993; OMB 1993a).

At the request of Congress, the Congressional Research Service explored research on using IT to simplify administration of health insurance claims, while the General Accounting Office began a study on implementation of automated medical record systems, and the OTA's Programs on Health and on Telecommunication and Computing Technologies undertook an extensive study on health care access, quality, and cost control using IT (OTA 1993a). The congressionally chartered but independent National Research Council, through its Computer Science and Telecommunications Board, began to consider how the NII could reduce the cost of health care and improve quality and access to services. Its earlier focus had been on internal issues such as data use and patient records.

Activity on linking digitized information to electronic networks also expanded in other federal departments. The Office of Disease Prevention and Health Promotion began an evaluation of a new Washington, DC–based electronic network of health and social service agencies intended to improve the coordination and effectiveness of community services (Public Health Service 1993). It also began planning for development of networked health information for the public in light of the NII and health care changes. Its National Health Information Center started a New Media unit to explore the potential of IT for public health information and education purposes (Office of Disease Prevention 1994).

A Blind Spot in the Visions

All of this executive, legislative, and evaluative activity provided the climate, direction, and resources to give a concerted thrust to an emerging, yet still unclear vision of the NII. These new efforts toward a civilian and civic society nonetheless continued to focus most resources on helping large-scale, sometimes conglomerate organizations adapt and renew themselves with IT to improve their performance in business and public service, health, education, information, and government. The unspoken assumption was that the public would benefit as recipients—not necessarily participants—by a kind of 'trickle-down' IT, and that somehow the more disadvantaged groups would have equitable gains.

Industry thought it was best suited to supply the structure and services, if the government would ensure a competitive electronic marketplace, picking up development and start-up costs and supplying funds where the market failed among disadvantaged groups. Public interest groups emphasized empowering a public that would not just be recipients of services—whether entertainment, commercial, or social—but would be initiatory and active, through an electronic civic infrastructure based on free and affordable universal access—one that would also allow disadvantaged individuals to join the digital mainstream, assuming they had access to usable technology.

Many of the NII proposed strategies included support structures. The administration's NII agenda called for developing manufacturing extension centers at local Small Business Administration offices to help businesses gain access to the new technologies and offer training to managers and workers in using them (Clinton and Gore 1993). It proposed interactive computer kiosks at federal centers around the country, such as the 1,300 Social Security offices, in which the public could communicate with federal agencies (NTIA 1993). Educational technology centers were designed to assist teachers and schools, and the federal library system (with its 1,400 depositories) would provide electronic support and assistance to researchers, educators, and advanced students. The midwestern higher educational institutions were expanding their support system, MIDNET, to help the transition to the NII and sustain an electronic environment. And the major public services were to be supported with funds to demonstrate the use of the NII, backed up by resources to design and evaluate new uses.

The White House itself, extending the electronic network the Clinton election campaign had used to communicate with its local units, established a public system through the Internet on which it sent speeches, press briefings, executive orders, and other documents to the public. And in 1993, Congress began a Constituent Electronic Mail System to interact with constitutents in each district.

All major constituencies, in other words, ranging from the general public to large businesses and nonprofit institutions, were to be supported with special resources to enter and help create the electronic future. All, that is, except small-scale, low-budget, community-based organizations in disadvantaged areas. Even the public interest groups, emphasizing the public good, conceived the public interest in individual terms, not having much awareness of the problems faced by low-income organizations that are part of the day-to-day lives of disadvantaged individuals—the day care, neighborhood, youth, and senior centers, the economic development offices and local housing advocates, the small community health and welfare providers, religious and secular. These provide needed services and are often bridges to wider services and resources. They are sometimes also the most informed and strongest advocates of the kinds of health-supporting changes that are urgently needed in their communities, but clearly have not been very successful. Their voices have not been heard.

If these groups are to be left at the side of the information highway, their voices will be still less articulate, less coherent and coordinated, less timely and less effective, as the rest of America moves beyond them. The gap between IT-rich and IT-poor communities means more than diminished access to information. It also means an impoverished capacity to build and broker services, to communicate with local and national sister groups, and to organize, mobilize, and effectively advocate for resources and accountability by public officials, their own representatives, and private economic enterprises. The national information infrastructure is part of the health-supporting infrastructure that is missing from disadvantaged communities and missing from the national vision of the NII.

References

Bass, G., and A. MacLean. 1993. "Enhancing the Public's Right to Know about Environmental Issues." *Villanova Environmental Law Journal* IV: 287–321.

Bass, G., and D. Plocher. 1989. "Strengthening Federal Information Policy: Opportunities and Realities at OMB." *Software Law Journal* 3 (3): 413–59.

Benton Foundation. 1994a. "The Communication Policy Project." Washington, DC: Benton.

———. 1994b. "Summary of Communications Legislation." Washington, DC, 10 June.

Bollier, D. 1993. "The Information Superhighway: Roadmap for Renewed Public Purpose." *Tikkun* (July/August): 20–22.

"Calling All Channels." 1993. *Business Week*, 27 September, 130–35.

Civille, R., M. Fidelman, and J. Altobello. 1993. *A National Strategy for Civic Networking: A Vision of Change*. Washington, DC: Center for Civic Networking.

Clinton, W., and A. Gore. 1993. *Technology for America's Economic Growth: A New Direction to Build Economic Strength*. Washington, DC: The White House, 22 February.

Committee on House Administration. 1993. *Government Printing Office Electronic Information Access Enhancement Act of 1993 Report*. Washington, DC: U.S. House of Representatives.

Committee on Rules and Administration. 1992. "GPO Gateway to Government Act of 1992," Senate 2813; "GPO Wide Information Network for Data Online Act of 1991," H.R. 2772. Prepublication Testimony. Washington, DC: U.S. Congress, 23 July.

Committee on Science, Space, and Technology. 1993. *National Information Infrastructure Act of 1993*. Report. Washington, DC: U.S. Congress.

Computer Professionals for Social Responsibility (CPSR). 1993. 21st Century Project. *Setting a New Course for Science and Technology Policy*. Palo Alto: CPSR.

———. 1994. "Serving the Community: A Public Interest Vision of the National Information Infrastructure." *CPSR Newsletter* 12 (1): 1–22.

Cooke, K., and D. Lehrer. 1993. "The Whole World is Talking." *Government Information Insider* (September/October): 4–6.

Corporation for Public Broadcasting (CPB). 1993. *Community-wide Education and Information Services Initiative*. Washington, DC: CPB.

Gore, A. 1993. *From Red Tape to Results: Creating a Government that Works Better and Costs Less*. Report of the National Performance Review. Washington, DC: The White House, 7 September.

Kapor, M., and J. Berman. 1993. "A Superhighway Through the Wasteland?" *New York Times*, 24 November, A15.

Lake, M. 1994. *What People Think About the New Communications Technologies*. Washington, DC: The Benton Foundation.

Love, J. 1992. *Information Policy for the Next Administrations*. Washington, DC: Center for the Study of Responsive Laws.

———. 1993a. "Information Policy for the Clinton/Gore Administration: A Viewpoint." *Government Publications Review* (20) 245–49.

———. 1993b. *A Review of the National Information Infrastructure*. Washington, DC: Taxpayer Assets Project.

McChesney, R. 1993. *Telecommunications, Mass Media, and Democracy: The Battle for the Control of U.S. Broadcasting, 1928–1935*. New York: Oxford University Press.

Morino Institute. 1994. *Assessment and Evolution of Community Networking*. Great Falls, VA: Morino Foundation.

National Telecommunications and Information Administration (NTIA). 1993. *The National Information Infrastructure: Agenda for Action*. Washington, DC: Department of Commerce, 15 September.

———. 1994. "Information Infrastructure Task Force." Washington, DC: U.S. Department of Commerce, 8 June.

Newman, T., et al. 1993. *Serving the Community: A New Grand Challenge. A Public Interest Vision of the National Information Infrastructure*. Draft. Washington, DC: Computer Professionals for Social Responsibility, 8 August.

Office of Disease Prevention and Health Promotion. 1994. "ODPHP Director's Report." Public Health Service. Washington, DC: DHHS, 1 January.

Office of Management and Budget (OMB). 1993a. *Management of Federal Information Resources*. OMB Circ. A-130. The White House, Washington, DC, 25 June.

———. 1993b. *Seminar on the National Information Infrastructure: Concept, Role of Government, and Preparing for the FY 1995 Budget*. Executive Office of the President, Washington, DC, 14 October.

———. 1993c. *Status of Pending Legislation*. Washington, DC: Executive Office of the President, 17 September.

Office of Technology Assessment (OTA). 1993a. *Information Technology and the Health Care System*. Washington, DC, U.S. Congress, October.

———. 1993b. *Wireless Technologies*. Washington, DC: U.S. Congress, November.

Public Health Service. 1993. *Community Services Network. Project Summary Report*. Washington, DC: U.S. Department of Health and Human Services.

Sirbu, M. 1992. "Telecommunication Technology and Infrastructure." In *Annual Review of the Institute for Information Studies 1992*, edited by C. Firestone. Aspen, CO: Aspen Institute.

Smarr, L., and C. Catlett. 1992. "Life after Internet." In *Building Information Infrastructure*, edited by B. Kahi. Cambridge, MA: Harvard Business School Press, 145.

Subcommittee on Science, Committee on Science, Space, and Technology. 1993. *High Performance in Computing and High Speed Networking Applications Act of 1993*. H.R. 1757. Washington, DC: U.S. House of Representatives, 27 April, 6 and 11 May.

Telecommunications Policy Roundtable. 1993. *Renewing the Commitment to a Public Interest Telecommunications Policy*. Press Release. Washington, DC: Center for Media Education, 26 October.

White House. 1993. *United States Advisory Council on the National Information Infrastructure*. Executive Order. Washington, DC, 15 September.

CHAPTER 16

EPILOGUE

Policy Prospects and Recommendations for Community Information Technology

IN THE fall of 1993, I faced responsible federal agencies and interest groups with questions about how out-of-the-mainstream organizations that are too poor to develop and sustain an information technology capacity would become part of the national information infrastructure. Virtually all said they had given the issue little, if any, attention. The only special groups that received explicit consideration were people with disabilities and some students in low-income schools (Subcommittee on Science 1993). The idea that disadvantaged people might receive better public services as a result of the NII, and that they as individuals should be afforded free or low-cost access to basic interactive services, was assumed but not well explored. No attention had been given in analyses, agendas, plans, policy, or legislation to build the IT capacity of small community-based organizations to enable them to quickly join the NII and strengthen their work in and with their communities or connect them to larger health and social agencies. This was a blind spot in the visions of the electronic future: there was no place for *community* information technology—IT infrastructure for IT-poor, community-based organizations that were often intermediaries between their local constituencies in poor areas and the resources that were otherwise beyond reach.

Public interest groups focused on information access by the public and the participation of the public in community and governmental decision making. They seemed to assume the degree of access to IT resources that middle and more-favored classes had or could be expected to have at their workplaces, libraries, schools, universities, and homes. The resource deficits faced by small community agencies and households were almost beyond their range of sight and experience.

Public interest groups were widely supportive of the idea of building IT capacity in disadvantaged community groups, once aware of the issues. They judged, however, that while some players in the current administration might be sympathetic to the idea, funds were not likely to be allocated. Congressional staff also agreed, saying that without explicit attention, statements about access for disadvantaged groups would remain rhetoric, as the annual funding for NII demonstrations would involve large-scale, profession-led service agencies that had no incentive to include low-budget, community-based organizations in their network planning. Academic experts from universities and research institutes who offered advice to the administration were concerned about the technical issues involved in developing the NII and ensuring competition among industry groups, but not about community IT.

Policy Perspective

The viewpoint that follows on national information infrastructure policy is drawn from the experiences described in previous chapters on IT used by and with disadvantaged communities to bind and build healthy communities. One theme runs through this book. Communities cannot be healthy without health-supporting infrastructures, including affordable housing, employment, education and training, environmental security, as well as basic health care. A new facet of that infrastructure is the IT capacity of community institutions that are able to inform and support the individuals they serve, deliver services, and advocate for community resources. They often form two-way bridges between residents and outside, large-scale government, corporate, and other organizations led by professionals.

Effective networked community coalitions and collaboration with sister communities and with public health and other agencies locally and nationally are necessary to obtain health-supporting resources in disadvantaged communities and brighten their prospects for health. But this will not be feasible in the foreseeable future unless IT capacity-building in those communities is explicit in NII policy development and is included in the reforms of health care and public health systems. Resource gaps will almost certainly grow if IT-rich and IT-poor organizations are tolerated at the policy level.

Community Strengths

As the stories of community IT showed, small, low-budget groups used IT as a way to deal with the growing gaps between the mushrooming problems they faced and available resources, as a set of new tools that might be effective and cost saving. They were not moved to action by the commercialized attractions of IT, but by real problems for which there seemed to be no more acceptable options. Even so, they faced an array of fiscal, technical, and political problems in developing and sustaining their IT programs, which supported aid to the homeless, after-school education for poor children, help for in-home caregivers, small business development, and other health-supporting activities.

They demonstrated a wider range of IT services and activities than is usually developed or discussed by business or public services groups, not only information and communication, but also organization development, community services delivery, advocacy, and mobilization. These community-based IT programs also reached a wider spectrum of users than is within the scope of commercial providers. These were user groups that also are often left unidentified, even when "the disadvantaged" are mentioned, but little discussed, in public policy forums (Gore 1993; National Coordinating Committee 1994; Brown 1993).

The cases of community IT also challenge the stereotype of the typical IT innovator or entrepreneur as being a young, white male "techie." The leadership in IT program development will now have to include women, the old and the young, majority and minority, those who are not "techies," and those who are skilled in and committed to the soft technologies of social organization and organization building.

Every community situation needed some sort of start-up system to begin its IT development, whether jerry-built or built into a parent organization in the form of financing and supplier networks, revenue streams and credit lines. These are support systems that large-scale organizations already have in place, along with decades of experience with conventional uses of computers. To the extent that the IT-poor community groups had to rely on potluck arrangements to start their programs, they were vulnerable to costly problems, like unscrupulous experts.

Yet in some communities, communitywide supports from public policies and investment had been made in incipient local IT infrastructure, through freenets, school and library IT programs, telecommuting incentives, and federal grants. These supports became inviting and valuable platforms from which to help launch the new IT ventures.

The low-budget groups often had to settle for a patchwork of IT support services, making it difficult to sustain their physical and human IT resources. None of their larger and better-endowed public and private counterparts—no business, university, school, hospital, library, or government agency—would initiate an IT program without an adequate backup system, as earlier chapters showed.

In the tangle of problems and uncertainties, these survivors found ways to meet their IT development problems, if tenuously and temporarily. Often their skills for doing so came intuitively, gained by long life in the community, both institutional and personal, and by trial and error, without the help of formal consultants, analysts, or lobbyists. The persistence, and sometimes courage, that they revealed stemmed from a commitment to making their communities better, healthier places. These qualities are invaluable resources of community life that could be more effective and multiplied if they were stimulated and supported by public policy in information technology, health, and other areas.

Bypassed

These vignettes revealed survivors. There is no way to know how many other stories would reveal efforts in community IT that were too hopeless to begin or that were tried and failed, even among groups with equal commitment but fewer resources. Left to the vagaries of the market, which places little value on "community" as social cohesion or as place, future survivors may find their IT programs shaped by the vision of an electronic shopping mall rather than as tools to build healthy communities.

For IT-poor organizations to avoid hitchhiker status, to avoid having to wait for some group to offer them, one by one, a ride on the information highway—but not a place at the policy negotiation table—will require the same degree of public commitment and support that has been made to more advantaged institutions in business, government, and profession-managed health, education, and social service organizations.

Federal policies recognize the need of *large* organizations for "organizational learning" and provide the resources to support it (IITF 1994). By including community-based groups in the digital mainstream at the outset, public policy could correct the design of the information highway, and also help mend the social fabric that divides and bodes ill for all of America's communities.

Public Accountability

One of the principle roles and responsibilities of government is to guide and ease the transition to the systemwide changes required by health care reform and the national information infrastructure, with special attention to ensuring equity among those whose voice is least articulated and least heard. That mission began to be acknowledged in policy-related papers of the Clinton administration, Congress, and public interest groups. Whether and how extensively and effectively the rhetoric produces changes on the ground in disadvantaged communities depends on the policy attention and resources that are committed to the effort—in a public arena of intense competition.

In the nine months after I initially raised the question with Washington officials about inclusion of IT-poor community organizations in the NII, many changes occurred that suggested at least small shifts in priorities and resource commitments that focus more attention not only on disadvantaged individuals, but on the local organizations that are part of their lives. The observations that follow derive from my participation in a few of the forums shaping the NII since my initial inquiry at the Office of Management and Budget, the Office of Technology Assessment, the Office of Disease Prevention and Health Promotion, the National Telecommunications and Information Administration, and other nongovernmental organizations.

Perhaps the strongest message about community information technology emerging from within the government came from OTA in its Congressional report *Making Government Work* (OTA 1993). It cautioned that many of the potential social benefits, including cost savings, of electronic delivery of government services through the NII would be lost if IT were not widely accessible, usable, and affordable. A *universal* NII required infrastructure development of not only IT hardware, but also development of the people and organizations that were already experienced in meeting the needs of local citizens and training and assisting them to use information and technology, like schools, libraries, community centers, town halls, and health agencies.

OTA recommended an "electronic public access safety net" and a partially federally funded nonprofit Corporation for Electronic Service Delivery, comparable to the Corporation for Public Broadcasting, to ensure ready access to public services. These information technology services could include federal cash and in-kind benefits transfer; information dissemination; grants, loans, and contracts transactions; citizen input in government processes; and job training.

To enable people's use of these services, OTA proposed that Congress have federal agencies use a small part of their budgets to involve citizens at the grass roots in developing IT access, to provide for community infrastructure development, and to create agency and government information directories—NII navigational tools—that are easy to use (OTA 1993).

Under the mandate of the administration's National Performance Review that sought to improve government efficiency through IT, and the goals of the NII Agenda for Action, some federal agencies modified their agendas and resource commitments (Gore 1993; Brown 1993). The National Library of Medicine within the National Institutes of Health, long a highly medically oriented and high technology–focused agency, initiated for the first time a grants program to enable selected types of community-based organizations to use IT. Funds covered the costs of IT, skills development, and information development and retrieval. The purposes were to improve information access for AIDS patients, their caregivers, and community agencies, including advocacy groups (NLM 1994).

Another "reengineering" process in the Department of Agriculture's Cooperative Extension Service gave birth to a Decisions for Health program through its 3,000 local sites. Projects were designed to bring together health care and educational institutions to strengthen community health care infrastructure by applying a variety of electronic technologies. They were to focus on disadvantaged communities and groups.

The Office of Disease Prevention and Health Promotion, following its mandate to provide health information to the public, began to explore changes in its methods in the light of the NII and health care reform. Initial issues dealt with information as a kind of thing unto itself, that is, how much and what kinds the public should get. Six months later greater attention was being given to community organizations and how they could be enabled to bridge the information and technology gap between the worlds of the IT haves and have-nots, especially in economically disadvantaged areas.

Another federal initiative, by volunteer staff from several cabinet departments, the White House, Congress, the Government Printing Office, and other governmental and private associations became Americans Communicating Electronically (ACE). ACE's focus was on access and participation for the Americans who did not own modems and computers, urging federal agencies to develop information access programs to foster "interactive citizen-government communications systems." ACE proposed to coordinate promotion of electronic, user-friendly, multiservice kiosks at the thousands of local federal government agency sites. In its initial volunteer efforts, ACE supplied selected federal documents to any user of the Internet within 48 hours, with personalized help for new users (White House 1993).

In the nongovernmental sector, in an effort to strengthen the voice of nonprofit and public interest groups in the NII policy arena, the Benton Foundation's Communications Policy Project set out to build this constituency into a cohesive force to advance policy options in support of the public interest. Unlike the discussion forum and volunteer nature of the Telecommunications Roundtable, the policy project had staff and program resources to support issue analyses, public education, and conferences—like the ones that helped propel development of the Center for Civic Networking and ACE.

Perhaps the strongest initiative favoring community information technology came from the small Bauman Foundation. Working with

OMB and other governmental agencies, foundations, public interest groups, and a wide spectrum of environmental and community-based social and economic development organizations, the foundation drafted a proposal for IT capacity-building in local nonprofit organizations. The goal was to enable these groups to use online governmental and other information and participate in community and public decision making. This would be done through partnerships between the government and philanthropic groups in developing support programs for "intermediary institutions to which the public turns for help"—public interest organizations, libraries, schools, and community-based groups, or other groups like community IT support centers (Bauman 1994). The types of support included federal responsibility for developing "information navigation" tools in software and print, training "information navigators" in service agencies and community groups, and funding the work of local groups that use online information to improve their communities.

In the months following the Public Interest Summit in 1994, described in Chapter 15, public interest groups were able to get measures introduced in several congressional committees that would prohibit "electronic redlining"—avoiding the fiber-optic cabling of poor neighborhoods—and ensure a "public right of way" on advanced telecommunications networks (Telecommunications Roundtable 1994). As important as these guarantees would be, they affected primarily those individual households able to afford computers and modems or cable TV systems. They would not build IT capacity in community organizations, although they would undergird the process.

The possibilities for organizational capacity-building came with demonstration grants administered by the National Telecommunications and Information Administration for which there were about 1,100 applications in the first year. The criteria for acceptance encompassed technical, hard technology issues and soft technology, social organization issues. These included equity of access to the electronic services by the public, especially disadvantaged groups, involvement of public and private representative groups in the planning and development processes, and means for ensuring benefits, such as training, ongoing support, and affordability, to targeted end-users (NTIA 1994).

Conceivably, the criteria encouraged community information technology, but most of the health-related proposals did not. The most polished proposals, not surprisingly, came from large-scale organizations accustomed to grant writing and most interested in high technology, such as telemedicine, medical imaging, and data transfer for health care providers and researchers. Few proposals came from state or local public health departments. Few included the general public, much less disadvantaged groups, as users or (even more rarely) as participants in IT system development. The few applications that most closely resembled community information technology and met the soft technology criteria were from IT-poor organizations, modest in size, with limited budgets, and not experienced in writing federal grant applications. They fared poorly in the winnowing process.

NII and Changes in Health Care

The legislation that would develop the NII and begin linking libraries, schools, government agencies, and health and social services had companion measures in the legislation on health care reform. Congressional measures hinted at a future that could offer new opportunities for collaboration through IT between health care, public health, and community-based organizations to improve the health of people in disadvantaged areas.

There were, for example, measures for new health promotion/disease prevention funds for "vulnerable groups" to examine health problems, undertake community-based action, and establish networks between public health agencies and the health care delivery system. Public health agencies would be responsible for providing information for consumers and providers of health care about preventive health services and the appropriate use of medical care, and for developing new public health prevention programs. New comprehensive school health programs would serve children of all ages, involve local health care providers and community-based organizations, and elicit broad-based community participation from parents, youth, and business leaders.

Public health and health care facilities were to use uniform data sets for monitoring community health and be connected by electronic networks. This would make possible IT linkages between providers, patients, and families in homes or nursing homes, thus increasing access by patients to their records and helping improve self-care and support for family caregivers.

Here again the image of the electronic future is mirrored on the past: IT enables providers to transmit their services to individuals as patients, consumers, and recipients. There is no provision for IT links with the community organizations as important collaborators. A fuller, more health-supporting vision, would incorporate community information technology, improving outreach, information and education services, training, planning, and coordination, and at the same time developing the strengths of local organizations. These possibilities were discussed earlier and seen in the case illustrations.

Local IT capacity-building and organizational development would serve the interests of effectiveness and efficiency of health care and public health agencies, while enabling local community groups—whether child care or senior centers, churches, libraries, community health centers, housing groups, or food banks—to serve their constituents more and better. It would move disadvantaged communities a step closer to being more health supporting, more like partners and providers than recipients and consumers, more like doers than "done to," empowering people beyond the resources of individual members.

Capacity-Building for IT-Poor Organizations in Disadvantaged Communities

Widespread development of community IT would require a national initiative led by federal policy, an initiative more explicit than appeared likely in the mid-1990s. This effort would call attention to the growing gap between IT-poor and IT-rich organizations as a new dimension of impoverishment in already disadvantaged communities and groups. A national policy would set goals and priorities for resource development, allocation, and action, and assign responsibility for follow-through and oversight to ensure the public interest in closing the gap in the NII, thus avoiding the customary "trickle down" hope for benefits at some future time. Such an achievement would be consistent with a strategy for community economic and social development, for building healthy communities.

Enabling Systems for Community Development: Community IT Support Centers

Because of the extensive IT deficits in the organizations of poor communities, IT support funds could create community IT support centers. These centers would be counterparts to those becoming available in more favored areas in schools, libraries, businesses, and as freestanding entities.

Preferably under the control of a local coalition of organizations, including small businesses, the support centers would develop IT capacity as organizational tools for community-based groups tailored to local needs. These first-stop, one-stop centers could provide a range of services directly or through local contracts whenever possible. The services might include technology transfer and liaison, demonstrating local relevance, providing public and media education, convening interested parties, and brokering organizational relationships to obtain needed resources. They would be catalysts for IT development and would be housed separately or as part of an appropriate community site, such as a library, church, neighborhood community development center, or educational institution (Milio 1993).

Information and Training

The IT support centers would act as sites for technology transfer, for information access, exchange, and dissemination. Among the types of information they would gather and reconfigure in community-friendly formats are databases on funders, model IT projects, sample documents such as grant applications, feasibility studies, bibliographic abstracts, and available local expertise among retirees, graduate school students, teachers, librarians, public service volunteers, and pro bono or low-cost consultants. These would be available on-line and in other customized formats through the center. Such resources would help local groups obtain the start-up and sustaining resources they need in the face of competition for public and private funds, an especially weighty problem for low-budget, small-scale organizations.

The centers would initially survey and inventory local IT needs and uses by public and private community-based organizations and small businesses. This in itself could be made a public education instrument about the uses and availability of IT. They would also offer public information sessions on-site and through local media on community uses of IT, showing its relevance to local activities and organizations.

They would train trainers for local groups' staff, hold workshops on IT program development and management issues, and encourage those experienced in community IT to share their on-the-ground knowledge with novices. Center staff would also provide consultant services to assist groups in developing strategic plans for community IT and convene IT experts and local groups to discuss, for example, collaborative design for IT software systems for local uses.

The IT centers would also be a resource for trouble-shooting, perhaps training community trouble-shooters who would volunteer to be available on-line to assist individuals and organizations with IT operating problems, including, by mutual agreement, doing the initial set-up of IT equipment. Retirees are untapped wealth in many communities, as the case studies showed.

Brokering

The problem of incompatible hardware for IT-novice organizations might be dealt with by collaboration among IT support centers to develop regional and local clearinghouses for recycling donor equipment that could be matched with the needs of small group users, a kind of halfway house for computers and software. Another way to ease the equipment problem is to broker arrangements between groups of local or regional sellers and buyers through bartering or very high discounts or donations in return for future sales and using the potential market power of a number of small-scale groups as joint buyers to obtain lower-cost, appropriate technology. Rewiring old facilities and adding dedicated telephone lines might also be addressed collectively by user groups and regional and national telecommunications corporations.

In these and the infinite number of other ways that local inventiveness always provides, IT support centers would bring technical information and skill to community groups. Further, through hands-on experience and training programs, they would also help transfer equally important program development and management know-how, and essential strategic skills like how to identify and develop wider interorganizational relations and respond to changes in organizational, political, and community environments. This would in turn prepare groups to participate in new networked relations as partners and providers of services, such as linking with local public health and other profession-managed agencies.

Planning and Development Grants

Beginning with a one-year collaborative planning process among local community groups, about five years of funding active IT support centers in disadvantaged communities should be enough to narrow the IT gap and wean the areas from the need for external hands-on IT support. Thereafter, they would have the capacity to use their IT skills to draw on the resources of the nation and the world.

Planning grant information should be widely distributed through local media and unique local sites, such as storefront churches, child care centers, and community development offices, in addition to the national umbrella groups that represent some of these community institutions.

Professional Education

Community IT should be further supported by federal funds to encourage classroom teaching in professional schools on "literacy in community IT"—how to work with communities that are adopting IT tools for services delivery and local development. Such courses should be included in basic and continuing education for health, education, and social service professionals—lawyers, public administrators, police, librarians, gerontologists, child care workers, and computer science students.

Modeling and Market Power

All levels of government should lead the way in community IT capacity-building by developing electronic relations with their decentralized units and partner organizations, and use their market power as large purchasers of IT to promote the most community-sensitive and user-friendly types. They should leverage their market power under public funds to encourage IT producers, ranging from telecommunications to software firms, to support IT capacity-building in less-advantaged local organizations.

Without specific priorities for structures and incentives for community IT where it is most needed, NII resources will bypass disadvantaged organizations in the minds and budgets of policymakers and service providers, and the gap between the IT-rich and IT-poor will widen, creating still less healthy communities.

A national community IT policy would stimulate and support a community-based IT infrastructure in the same way that vast federal sums have done for large-scale, corporate purposes for decades. Creating enabling systems for small scale organizations in disadvantaged areas would build an IT infrastructure at the grass roots that offers more fertile ground for healthier, cohesive communities, and would be consistent with the goals for the national information infrastructure, public health, and health care reform. Widening the vision of the electronic future and enabling it to work in disadvantaged areas will provide new tools to help rebuild hope for a healthier America.

References

Bauman, P. 1994. "Capacity-Building: A Partnership for Government and the Non-Profit Sector." Draft. Washington, DC: The Bauman Foundation, 9 May.

Brown, R. 1993. *The National Information Infrastructure: Agenda for Action*. Washington, DC: U.S. Department of Commerce, September.

Gore, A. 1993. *Creating a Government that Works Better and Costs Less*. The Report of the National Performance Review. Washington, DC: The White House, September.

Information Infrastructure Task Force (IITF). 1994. "What It Takes to Make It Happen: Key Issues for Applications of the National Information Infrastructure." Committee on Applications and Technology. Gaithersburg, MD: U.S. Department of Commerce, 25 January.

Milio, N. 1994. "Community IT: Capacity-Building for IT-Poor Organizations in Disadvantaged Communities." Policy Seminar on the National Information Infrastructure, Executive Office of the President, Washington, DC, 14 October.

National Coordinating Committee on Technology in Education and Training, the National Information Infrastructure. 1994. "Requirements for Education and Training." Washington, DC, 25 March.

National Library of Medicine (NLM). 1994. "Statement of Work: AIDS Information Outreach Projects." Washington, DC: National Institutes of Health.

National Telecommunications and Information Administration (NTIA). 1994. "Availability of Funds." Washington, DC: U.S. Department of Commerce, March.

Office of Technology Assessment (OTA). 1993. *Making Government Work: Delivery of Government Services*. Washington, DC: U.S. Congress, November.

Subcommittee on Science, Committee on Science, Space and Technology. 1993. *Hearings H.R. 1757. High Performance Computing and High Speed Networking Applications Act of 1993. April 27, May 6, 11.* Washington, DC: U.S. House of Representatives.

Telecommunications Roundtable. 1994. "Ninety-three Groups Press Congress for Right-of-Way on Information Highway." Press Release. Washington, DC, 12 May.

White House. 1993. "The Development of a Communications Network Program between the Federal Government and the American Public." Washington, DC: The White House, December.

APPENDIX

A Note on Framework and Method

Approach and Purpose

This book is based on detailed case studies in community information technology and the relevance they have for public policy. The policy aspect was developed through extensive interviews with federal policy officials and document analysis. The purpose was to try to understand what kinds of processes and problems organizations in poor communities face in developing their information technology capacity, to draw policy implications from these findings, and then to assess the feasibility of policy support for information technology capacity-building in the current federal policy environment. As discussed in the text (Chapter 4), information technology can provide new tools to support the development of healthy communities in direct and more subtle but crucial ways, improving access to health information and services on one hand and creating health-supporting community resources such as education and housing on the other.

Analytic Framework

The working proposition used for the information technology case and policy studies is that a program or policy issue, whether in an organization in a community or in Washington, D.C., draws the attention of public and private groups that view a prospective program or policy change as important to their interests. This occurs within an enabling or a restrictive social context (Burkhardt and Brass 1990). These stakeholders deploy their resources to influence the shape, pace, or direction of change in ways that either will enhance or at least will not harm their interests. Their effectiveness depends on their influence, status, resources, and skill compared with competing groups. The interplay among these organized units determines whether, to what extent, and in what form a program or policy moves through various phases from initiation to adoption, implementation, and beyond (Milio 1988, 1990; Rochefort and Cobb 1993).

Stakeholders

The aim of this inquiry was to trace community information technology programs from the idea phase to implementation by the initiating organizational unit, known variously as the "idea champion," the "sponsor," the focal or parent organization, or the "keeper" (Galbraith 1982; Milio 1988). This decision trail is seen as a negotiating or political process (Dorff and Steiner 1987) among organized stakeholders (parties at interest), whether represented by elected or bureaucratic officials (Feldstein 1988; Weller 1980), commercial (Bergthold 1990), scientific or medical (Austin and Overholt 1988; Warner 1991), or voluntary nonprofit entities (DiMaggio and Anheier 1990). Each stakeholder tries to enhance its interests—that is, to advance its agenda, which is derived from whatever is necessary to its survival and growth. Usually, survival means satisfying its own supporters (board, funders, bureaucratic superiors, membership, clientele, collaborators, and potential supporters) in a manner that they approve (Hord 1986) and in ways that at least sustain the legitimacy of the organization, if not also bringing influence and expansion (Alter and Hage 1992).

Stakeholders (or interest groups) are those groups whose interests are or are perceived by themselves to be affected by a change in program or policy. These *interests* include funds, facilities, staff, authority, control, status, and legitimacy, all of which affect a group's current and future bargaining power (Knoke 1989). Having hard assets usually confers an image of effectiveness, which in turn makes bargaining for more resources easier. Organized groups that are small, new, minimally resourced, and "different" in their aims have problems starting up and surviving (Yutchman and Seashore 1967; Minkoff 1993).

Stakeholder actions are based on a group's judgment of the "best" program or policy solution in light of its perception of a problem of social relevance (e.g., delivery of housing, health, or information services) or of organizational relevance (e.g., limits on advocacy). Organizations that view their interests to be at stake in a given situation will act to secure a pace and direction of change that they judge will enhance their interests—conditioned by their view of other urgent organizational priorities, potential costs and gains of action or inaction, and the resources they can commit to the action task, including funds, staff, skill, time, and access to information and decision makers.

Processes

The framework views program development (e.g., a new community IT program) and policymaking (e.g., a new policy to support community IT) as continuous social and political processes that, for simplicity, may be divided into phases: initiation (the idea), adoption (decision to undertake), implementation (on-the-ground activation), evaluation (assessment of results), and reformulation (to alter or rescind) (Milio 1988; Rochefort 1993). The processes are linked in all phases to a history and are not necessarily linear in their movement nor confined to formal procedures.

The *initiation* phase is viewed as including such processes as awareness by an affected group(s) of the importance of the issue (e.g., of developing an IT program or policy), defining and delimiting the problem in more specific terms, and determining whether it is a legitimate one for the group to address (Goodman 1987). The group, whether a formal organizational unit or not, next must decide the priority that it will accord the problem as an item for action, thus determining the resources it is willing to allocate or develop for its solution (Basch 1984). Then follows the design of acceptable options for action and choosing the course to pursue (Parcel, Simons-Morton, and Kolbe 1988). For our purposes, this means the adoption of a community IT program or policy as a way to strengthen local resources for improving the health and well-being of disadvantaged communities.

The "options for action" include substantive questions such as the shape of the IT program, and strategic issues, such as which stakeholders to involve and when and how to develop resources for implementation (Monahan and Scheirer 1988; McCarthy and Zald 1973). The *implementation* phase establishes the program using similar negotiating processes with parties at interest—for example, fiduciaries, funders, contractors (information service providers, packagers, carriers, equippers), employees, collaborators, competitors, and clients.

Evaluation is mainly nonformal, involving the perceived or explicit satisfaction of important constituencies (Brewer and De Leon 1983). Scientific evaluation, when it is done, is rarely if ever a direct or overriding influence in the decision to continue or end a program (Brint 1990; Whitman 1985).

Strategic Issues

Planning strategic actions to propel movement from idea to on-the-ground reality requires measures that will enhance the feasibility of the program. The program must be made economically feasible to its supporters and users, politically acceptable to the more powerful groups affected by it, socially acceptable within the milieu in which it is to operate, and administratively possible (Milio 1988). This involves searches for and obtaining resources and the effective and timely organization of resources to reach program development goals while maintaining essential intergroup linkages.

The *capacity* of an organization to influence these program and policy decisions depends mainly on its resources, age, size, and authority or prestige in the hierarchy (or hierarchies) of groups with which it must deal (Milio 1986; Useem and Zald 1987). It also must be able to use its resources skillfully. This means being able to acquire and develop timely and pertinent information ("intelligence") and employ it with the degree of aggressiveness required, ranging from passive uses (monitoring, analyzing, evaluating, reporting, or critiquing an issue) to more active ones (informing, educating, persuading, mediating, activating, or mobilizing others to act) (Lindblom and Cohen 1979).

The organization must use the most useful *types of information* (i.e., the types relevant and credible to each of its target groups), choosing among a spectrum of hard (factual, systematically gathered) data and soft (interpretations, opinions) forms. Science and verifiable, hard information has rarely been decisive or even persuasive in organizational negotiations about program or policy development (Brint 1990). Although science data are often used, the purpose is almost always strategic: to justify choices that are determined on a political, that is, negotiated, basis with trade-offs between the major stakeholders in a particular situation (Brewer and De Leon 1983; Laumann and Knoke 1987).

A stakeholder, whether the parent or a target organization, must also decide the tenor of the information it will use—that is, whether as incentive or veiled threat. Finally, the organization decides the most effective channels through which to convey its message, whether directly to the target group or by indirect means, ranging from mediators (influentials), to public opinion formation, to public demonstrations and the use of the professional or mass media (Milio 1990).

Organizations relate to each other on a voluntary or mandated basis, and through ad hoc or formalized arrangements, any of which may be affected by personal (as opposed to impersonal) ties among the individuals involved (Cohen 1992). The sets of relations influence the essential bargaining nature of the interactions, resulting in varying degrees of influence over decisions about resources, cooperation, coordination, or conflict. This climate then affects the feasibility of effective program development and implementation (Tessler and Goldman 1982; Schermerhorn 1975; Gray 1989).

Method

This inquiry into community information technology—which at this writing has been virtually unexplored in disadvantaged community organizations—meets generally accepted criteria for using the case study as its chief method: contemporary phenomena set in historical, evolving contexts, composed of "non-events" and processes over which the outsider has no control, and requiring many sources of evidence (Yin 1989; Guess and Farham 1989). This approach can obtain the kind of information needed to develop interpretations and understanding, to derive "lessons" or "working rules of thumb" (rather than primarily to explain or test theory). The method also, in this instance, can help those who are unacquainted with the possibilities of community information technology to envision it in a practical sense. This is intended to make the material more useful and credible to potential users, whether practitioners or policymakers, and help focus attention toward small-scale, community users and uses that support strengthening communities and promoting people's well-being and health (Brewer and De Leon 1983; MacRae 1989; Whitman 1985).

Research findings are used very little by decision makers (Beyer and Trice 1982; Webber 1987). The results apparently must first be made relevant to organizational or political priorities (Johnson 1985; McClintock 1987). Only in recent years are public health researchers and practitioners again becoming aware of the importance of working more closely with policymakers and the public in order to implement their findings (Stivers 1991). This political reality called for the second aspect of this work, an effort to assess the feasibility of policy support for community information technology among relevant federal officials, to take account of their perspectives and the policy environment in which they are working as a means to draw attention to community information technology and its implications for community well-being.

Site Selection

The case study sites were chosen to illuminate the problems and strategies of developing community information technology in contrasting settings, diverse populations, and variations in community IT. The small number of cases, although not uncommon (Thomas 1994; Marshall and Rossman 1989), was more limited than initially planned because of time and cost constraints. Completing the project required a six-month sabbatical and several small but critical grants.

The particular sites were initially selected from a computerized literature search, and an earlier pilot study based on a mail survey and site interviews, as well as informal, word-of-mouth sources. The site visits and interviews (including the policy study) took place between December 1991 and October 1993, and lasted from three days to two weeks each, depending on the availability of the interviewees and the complexity of the situation. All but three of the interviews were face-to-face and lasted about 90 minutes on average, usually between 45 and 75 minutes. The other three interviews were conducted by telephone.

Informants and Interviews

Informants were selected after telephone and written exchanges with the site organization over a period of weeks or months, obtaining written material on its community IT and general programs, its willingness to have a site visit at an agreed time, and arrangements for appointments with interviewees, each of whom was individually contacted.

The informants were individuals initially selected on the basis of the previsit information and in line with the conceptual approach to the cases—that is, stakeholders (the organizations that affected or were affected by the community IT venture)—and through a "snowball" process on advice from on-site informants. The organizational officials were those who had some degree of discretionary authority over the resources of their organizational unit and could speak for that unit, beyond any personal opinions they may have had. In all there were 77 in the case studies, ranging from 7 in Midcity to 22 in Indy, and 18 in the policy study. In addition, 108 policy-oriented people were involved in the Washington-based forums I participated in after October 1993 (Chapter 16).

The *interviews* were semistructured and focused on the initiation, implementation, and maintenance of the IT programs. They included exploration of the processes involved, the problems faced and how they were dealt with (especially resource issues), and a description of the IT program itself and any attempt at evaluating its impact. The interviews also covered, from the viewpoint of the informant, the background of the organization, why it became involved with the program, what it hoped to gain, and finally, a review of the chronology of events in the history of the IT venture and expectations about its future. In the policy study, the focus was on current policies in various phases of development, exploration into whether anything resembling support for community IT was being given attention, and if not, whether such support was likely or possible in the future.

I was familiar with much of this information before going to the sites. I had requested a variety of reports from the numerous organizations involved in each case, as well as independent sources of data on the local community and state, such as U.S. population, socioeconomic, and health-related data. In addition, I obtained, usually on-site, archival information in the form of memos, reports, planning documents, fiscal data, computer printouts, and newspaper clippings. In the policy study, I used legislation, printed congressional hearings, and a variety of policy reports and assessments from governmental and other sources, which I had obtained over several years. These provided the background for the face-to-face queries.

Confidentiality

Informants were assured of strict confidentiality of their person and, in the case studies, of their organization and jurisdiction. Fictitious names are used in the case descriptions below the regional or multistate level. Otherwise, all data—socioeconomic, political, health-related, and institutional—are site-specific and empirical. Quoted and noncited material in the text is drawn mainly from the interviews, with a few from written sources that are not cited to avoid identifying the site.

Data Collection and Analysis

This is a series of qualitative studies using guided interviews as the main channel for gathering information. The analyses were constructed around interpretations of the perceptions of key players—the stakeholder organizations—the paper trail of the case, and contextual information on the environment in which the organizations were operating.

The unit of analysis is the organization or organizational unit (e.g., agency, center, business, department, bureau)—one having a degree of discretionary control over a portion of organizational resources. The reason for using the organization rather than individuals as the focus of attention is that individuals in organizations are dispensable when they are out of tune with organizational priorities. In addition, individuals cannot carry out organizational purposes without support. Even the best-educated and most technologically aware professionals, for example, need more than information about IT to adopt and adapt to it, to go through the effort to reinvent it for their purposes. For this, they need organizational support—resources, ongoing training, technical backup, and assurances that IT will not threaten their job status (Backer 1987; Brown 1987; AHCPR 1992; Schmitz and Fuld 1991). Thus, *organizations*—individuals acting in their authoritative positions in organizations—redirect resources in ways that can change organizational operations, thereby affecting clienteles, constituencies, consumers, and communities.

Once arranged into a coherent picture from the variety of information sources, the material on each case was combed for the community IT developmental issues and problems faced over time, the stakes involved for participating organizations, the strategies used to move forward, the unanticipated impacts, the common threads among the cases, and the policy implications of the experiences (Tesch 1990; Altheide 1987; Strauss and Corbin 1990).

Study Limitations

All studies, qualitative and quantitative alike, have their limitations, of course. Case studies, on their face, are thought not to meet the conventional test of being scientific because they are too close to individual experience and have too many variables. Case studies therefore deal with variables as wholes rather than selecting a few to study, as quantitative studies do (that narrowness, too, can skew the view of reality or "truth"). Case studies are limited in time and space, as are statistical analyses, but *analytic* descriptions of cases can produce "so what" results. We can draw understandings and wider meaning, including testable propositions, from the complex experiences described in case studies (Bailey 1992). Case studies also have the potential to produce valuable information about the richness of human experience and provide images and insights that can be heuristic devices for both on-the-ground practitioners and organizations and policymakers.

The use of many data *sources*—internal and external to the organizations involved in the cases, written and verbal, formal, public, and nonformal—strengthens the validity of the collected information, and is known as triangulation (Patton 1990; Sandelowski 1986; Miles and Huberman 1984). The *type* of informant is also important. Informants were selected based on their organizations and their positions, having responsibility and discretionary authority with respect to the community information technology program; they could provide contrasting, sometimes nonsupportive perspectives on events. This diversity added to the validity of the studies and enriched the picture of the complex processes of organizational change—which cannot be captured by discrete quantitative data. Where views about factual information conflicted, these were followed up and checked in the archival documents and through third parties (i.e., by triangulation).

Although the informants were generous in their time and apparent willingness to present their views, some may have been reluctant to say more than they did, and not all relevant stakeholders may have been contacted. All of those who were contacted, however, agreed to an appointment, with one exception in the policy study. Face-to-face interviewing in the natural context of the informant, as compared with questionnaire surveys, usually improves cooperation, allows greater depth, the exploration of interconnections among important issues, and clarification of views, and can assist with finding other key informants and obtaining useful documents. This improves the accuracy—the reliability—of the findings.

Using many sources of convergent evidence, interlinking and comparing them, and placing them within the chronological and archival information framework all added to the validity of the studies and improved the reliability of the material. Reliability is also strengthened by having a single interviewer using a similar line of questions within the relatively short period of about 18 months (Kraemer et al. 1989).

The nature of case studies makes replication difficult as a means to assure validity, and misinterpretation of the data is always possible. However, these problems can be controlled by giving the reader the author's "pair of glasses" for viewing the information and describing the context and process of the work, as this and other sections of the book attempt to do. The methods in these case studies allowed verification by triangulation: cross-checking information among informants through in-depth interviews and with official documents, and using a guiding framework that required contact with potential nonsupporters of the IT programs.

While the case findings in themselves may not be widely applicable, the comparison of cases and breadth of selection will allow useful program inferences to be drawn through the analysis of real-world experience. This provides a basis for the development of plausible options for program and policy. Whatever the limits, it is doubtful that the information obtained here to inform health-supporting policy and program development could be usefully obtained without using on-the-ground methods (Brewer and De Leon 1983).

References

Agency for Health Care Policy and Research (AHCPR). 1992. *Information Dissemination to Health Care Practitioners and Policymakers*. Rockville, MD: U.S. Public Health Service, April.

Alter, C., and J. Hage. 1992. *Organizations Working Together: Coordination in Interorganizational Networks*. Newbury Park, CA: Sage Publications.

Altheide, D. 1987. "Ethnographic Content Analysis." *Qualitative Sociology* 10 (1): 65–67.

Austin, J., and C. Overholt. 1988. "Nutrition Policy: Building the Bridge Between Science and Politics." *Annual Review of Nutrition* 8: 1–20.

Backer, T. 1987. "Research Utilization and Managing Innovation in Rehabilitation Organizations." *Journal of Rehabilitation* 54 (2): 18–22.

Bailey, M. 1992. "Do Physicists Use Case Studies? Thoughts on Public Administration Research." *Public Administration Review* 52 (1): 11–14.

Basch, C. 1984. "Research on Disseminating and Implementing Health Education Programs in Schools." *Journal of School Health* 54: 57–66.

Bergthold, L. 1990. *Purchasing Power in Health, Business, the State, and Health Care Politics*. New Brunswick, NJ: Rutgers University Press.

Beyer, J., and H. Trice. 1982. "The Utilization Process: A Conceptual Framework and Synthesis of Empirical Findings." *Administrative Science Quarterly* 27: 591–622.

Brewer, G., and P. De Leon. 1983. *Foundations of Policy Analysis*. Homewood, IL: Dorsey.

Brint, S. 1990. "Rethinking the Policy Influence of Experts: From General Characterizations to Analysis of Variation." *Sociological Forum* 5 (3): 361–85.

Brown, B. 1987. "Networking Between Research and Service Delivery." *International Journal of Addictions* 22 (4): 310–17.

Burkhardt, M. E., and D. J. Brass. 1990. "Changing Patterns or Patterns of Change: The Effects of a Change in Technology on Social Network Structure and Power." *Administrative Science Quarterly* 35: 104–27.

Cohen, P. 1992. *Interorganization Coalitions: Assessing Effectiveness*. Paper presented at the American Public Health Association Annual Meeting, Washington, DC, 10 November.

DiMaggio, P., and H. Anheier. 1990. "The Sociology of Non-profit Organizations and Sectors." *Annual Review of Sociology* 16: 137–59.

Dorff, R., and J. Steiner. 1987. "Decision Cases in Western Democracies." *Comparative Political Studies* 20: 160–73.

Feldstein, P. J. 1988. *The Politics of Health Legislation: An Economic Perspective*. Ann Arbor, MI: Health Administration Press.

Galbraith, J. 1982. "Designing the Innovating Organization." *Organization Dynamics* (Winter): 5–25.

Goodman, R. 1987. "Factors Affecting Long Term Viability of Health Promotion Programs." Ph.D. Dissertation, University of North Carolina, Chapel Hill.

Gray, B. 1989. *Collaborating: Finding Common Ground for Multiparty Problems*. San Francisco: Jossey-Bass.

Guess, A., and P. Farham. 1989. *Cases in Public Policy Analysis*. New York: Longman.

Hord, S. M. 1986. "A Synthesis of Research on Organizational Collaboration." *Educational Leadership* (February): 22–26.

Johnson, K. 1985. "Research Influence in Decisionmaking to Control and Prevent Violence." *Knowledge* 7 (2): 161–89.

Knoke, D. 1989. "Resource Acquisition and Allocation in U.S. National Associations." *International Social Movement Research* 2: 129–54.

Kraemer, K. L., L. King, N. E. Dunkle, and J. P. Lane. 1989. *Managing Information Systems: Change and Control in Organizational Computing*. San Francisco, London: Jossey-Bass, xv–97.

Laumann, E., and D. Knoke. 1987. *The Organizational State*. Madison, WI: University of Wisconsin Press.

Lindblom, C., and D. Cohen. 1979. *Usable Knowledge*. New Haven, CT: Yale University Press.

MacRae, D. 1989. "Policy Analysis and Research Utilization." Paper presented at the Association for Public Policy Analysis and Management, Arlington, VA, 2–4 November.

Marshall, C., and G. Rossman. 1989. *Designing Qualitative Research*. London: Sage.

McCarthy, J., and M. Zald. "The Trend of Social Movements in America: Professionalization and Resource Mobilization." In M. Zald and J. McCarthy (eds.). 1973. *Social Movements in an Organizational Society,* 337–91. Chicago: Transaction Press.

McClintock, C. 1987. "Administrators as Information Brokers: A Managerial Perspective on Naturalistic Evaluation." *Evaluation and Program Planning* 10: 315–23.

Miles, M., and A. Huberman. 1984. *Qualitative Data Analysis*. Beverly Hills, CA: Sage.

Milio, N. 1986. "Pressure Groups and Australian Health Policymaking in the 1980s." *Politics* (November): 51–61.

———. 1988. "Making Healthy Public Policy: Learning the Science by Observing the Art. An Ecological Model for Policy Studies." *Health Promotion International* 2 (3): 35–54.

———. 1990. *Nutrition Policy for Food-Rich Countries: A Strategic Analysis*. Baltimore, MD: Johns Hopkins University Press.

Minkoff, D. 1993. "The Organization of Survival: Women's and Racial-Ethnic Voluntarist and Activist Organizations, 1955–1985." *Social Forces* 71 (June): 887–908.

Monahan, J., and M. Scheirer. 1988. "The Role of Linking Agents in the Diffusion of Health Promotion Programs." *Health Education Quarterly* 15 (4): 17–22.

Parcel, G., B. Simons-Morton, and L. Kolbe. 1988. "School Health Promotion: Integrating Organizational Change and Student Learning Strategies." *Health Education Quarterly* 15 (4): 25–39.

Patton, M. 1990. *Qualitative Evaluation Methods*. Beverly Hills, CA: Sage.

Rochefort, D., and R. Cobb. 1993. "Problem Definition, Agenda Access, and Policy Choice." *Policy Studies Journal,* 21 (1): 56–71.

Sandelowski, M. 1986. "The Problem of Rigor in Qualitative Research." *Advances in Nursing Science* 8, 27–37.

Schermerhorn, J. R. 1975. "Determinants of Interorganizational Cooperation." *Academy of Management Journal* 18 (December): 846–56.

Schmitz, J., and J. Fuld. 1991. "Organizational Colleagues, Media Richness, and Electronic Mail: A Test of the Social Influence Model of Technology Use." *Communication Research* 18 (4): 487–523.

Stivers, C. 1991. "The Politics of Public Health: The Dilemma of a Public Profession." In T. Litman and S. Robins (eds.). *Health Politics and Policy,* 356–69. Albany, NY: Delmar.

Strauss, A., and J. Corbin. 1990. *Basics of Qualitative Research*. Newbury Park, CA: Sage.

Tesch, R. 1990. *Qualitative Research.* London: Sage.

Tessler, R., and H. Goldman. 1982. *The Chronically Mentally Ill: Assessing Community Support Programs*. Cambridge, MA: Ballinger.

Thomas, R. 1994. *What Machines Can't Do*. Berkeley: University of California Press.

Useem, M., and M. Zald. 1987. "From Pressure Group to Social Movement." *Social Movements in an Organizational Society* (Special Issue).

Warner, K. 1991. "Tobacco Industry Scientific Advisors: Serving Society or Selling Cigarettes?" *American Journal of Public Health* 81 (7): 839–42.

Webber, D. J. 1987. "Factors Influencing Legislators' Use of Policy Information and Implications for Promoting Greater Use." *Policy Studies Review* 6 (4): 64–80.

Weller, P. 1980. "Determinants of Canadian Health Policy." *Journal of Health Politics, Policy, and Law* 5 (3): 405–18.

Whitman, D. 1985. "The Fate of Policy Analysis in Congressional Decision Making." *Western Political Science Quarterly* 38 (2): 294–311.

Yin, R. 1984. *Case Study Research*. London: Sage.

———. 1989. *Case Study Research: Design and Methods*. Newbury Park, CA: Sage.

Yuchtman, E., and S. Seashore. 1967. "A System Resource Approach to Organizational Effectiveness." *American Sociological Review* 32: 891–903.

INDEX

ABOUT THE AUTHOR

Nancy Milio is Professor of Health Policy and Administration (School of Public Health) and Professor of Nursing at the University of North Carolina at Chapel Hill. She received her Ph.D. in Sociology at Yale University. Her teaching, research, and writing focus on policy development, implementation, and evaluation; health policy and strategic analysis; community information technology; and health promotion and education. She has worked for 20 years as a policy analyst and consultant with the World Health Organization and with numerous governments including Scandinavia, Eastern and Western Europe, China, and Australia. She was involved in community organization for health during the 1960s. Among her seven published books are: *9226 Kercheval: The Storefront That Did Not Burn*, *The Care of Health in Communities: Access for Outcasts*, *Promoting Health Through Public Policy*, and *Nutrition Policy for Food-Rich Countries*. She has also published over 100 articles in 40 health, social science, and policy journals in seven countries. She has been a visiting professor at universities in the United Kingdom, New Zealand, Australia, The Netherlands, Spain, and Brazil.